About the Author

James Robert Clark, an initiate of the 9th circle, has studied under several Masters including Paul Twitchell, Harold Klemp, Michael Owen, and others.

He became deeply involved in spirituality after attending a lecture at the U of Delaware on spiritual awareness in 1971 and for the first time, hearing about out of body experiences. Then he read Paul Twitchell's book, "The Key to Secret Worlds," that he bought in a book store on the topic.

He has written many books as listed in the bibliography that teach Spirituality and related topics including: Healing, Health, Longevity and Quantum Vibrations.

He holds a BAS in art from U of D and a professional degree in architecture from Boston Architectural College and was first registered in 1983. He is a practicing registered professional Architect and Planner with projects in several states, but mainly Delaware, Maryland, and Virginia. Is an inventor with two US patents.

Interests and hobbies include, Painting, Figure Drawing, Ceramic Sculpture, Woodworking and Furniture Design, Sailing, Tennis, Flying, Boatbuilding, Fishing, Skiing, Sports Car Restoration, and Gardening.

The Dirt on Aging
7/26/18

by James Robert Clark, Architect/ Planner

Dedication

This book is dedicated to all of those people out there who have worked so very hard to stay trim and well, but have been lied to by the FDA sponsored drug companies and professionals that they trust. My hope here is that I have helped to get this useful message across with my books... that you are in control and these uniformed experts can no longer take charge of your life.

Forward:

Please follow me as I lead you back on this ancient path to wellness, health, antiaging, and joy long abandoned after thousands of years in pursuit of industrialization and its promise of easier living. Today, we sacrifice even more, as we focusing on cool gadgets, convenience, and quantity, at all cost. But we are paying a heavy price for all of this, as I point out herein and others reinforce in their talks herein.

A good bit of this payment includes having our life spans and lives defined by unwritten established government limits that bear little resemblance to the actual conditions that affect our health and with them, our quality of life.

Thus, this book is about re-adapting our abandoned ancient lifestyles, nutritional and otherwise. that few even considered in the past or recognize today. Interestingly, this nutritional pathway is again opened up and made possible in this age of consumer computer shopping and the availability of high quality dense foods and the many ancillary supplements discussed herein. These allow those of us made aware to make an end run around the key problems that got us here. So these high quality foods, once unavailable or even known to us only twenty years ago are now accessible and even sold online competitively.

With the above, along with adding a little creative gardening skills on our own, and the current science not available to the masses, as documented here that I point out, we can reestablish new life extending eating and living habits across the board

While the vibrations in the form of Sound and Light have always been available, all along. These vibratory elements have often been suppressed for quite some time by the mainstream. Now, we can augment our diets with superior quality, dense foods and supplements in what we now consider developed countries where diets are currently woefully deficient, especially in the US, but also in the highly regarded Mediterranean countries where people still only live a few years longer than the US.

In order to do this, you must first recognize that the mass media forces in control are constantly feeding us bogus facts that can and must kill us over time when adapted in many aspects of our lives, but especially nutritionally. By simply adapting these countermeasures, you are on the road to antiaging and wellness. Few, if anyone, speaks of them elsewhere and you are certainly not going to hear any of this from a reporter or professional on your daily news program. What you will hear about there is the very complex set of interactive systems that typically fails when it is not supplied with this simple set of measures offered herein. The result is that you live many more years than is even envisioned by people now.

Following The Dirt, An Interactive Journey:

- The Format/ Ground Rules for this book.
- Suggested method of reading the attached Videography/ web information.
- How to reference and most effectively use this video information.

Video/web references have extensively appeared in my books since, "It's the Liver Stupid," the first, now in its 5th edition, when I first initiated this format. This written/ video format has somewhat changed and expanded over this some fifteen year or so period, when I first introduced it in Yahoo Groups. This is especially true since a great deal of the current related science was unavailable then. Today, some of it is readily available on You Tube. They appear more on some of my recent books along with my own presentations and with those that that others have recommended as well as my own discoveries.

Today, most any topic, whether mainstream or radically controversial is offered in You Tube lectures. The author has also included much of his work, especially Dr. Price and my experimentation there, but also references are used to help defend these controversial emerging breakthroughs. Furthermore, at times, You Tube lectures cover a few significant, ground breaking, yet unpublished discoveries that others have recently proven, but have not cleared via peer review. This, with my discoveries, is the meat of my books. First, I dowse the lecture content. If it passes, I report it. My dowsing, "post event line," tests at nearly 100% accurate, but you decide.

Finally, if little of the rest of the remaining video is significant in itself, but one key point serves to establish something that the author sees as a key reference, the beginning point of that reference is noted in parenthesis i.e. (34:00). So this indicates that the key reference point is 34 minutes into the video. Further, if there are several other key points in an otherwise less relevant video, those will be noted following the first to save you time. In every case, the author has viewed the entire presentation at least once. Rarely, a video is used multiple times with multiple references to establish other key points.

Keep in mind that books will always outlast You Tube video references and you may have to reestablish any links lost yourself unless a newer edition is published. The attempt here is to provide enough information to do that, but it is impossible.

Interestingly, the first edition of "It's the Liver Stupid," has almost no live links left. Many have been lost or have changed within just the past few years as You Tube updates.

This "The Dirt on Aging" actually uses this format less often than previous books, simply because there is little actual video content reported on the topics today. That is, it is virtually new territory in many ways to lecturers, but they are also considered mundane and proven. I have found few web references on these topics, unlike my earlier books, even though you commonly hear related conversations every day and aspects are often discussed in everyday conversations if you are paying attention.

To use the few links provided effectively, you must be at least have a handheld computer or cell handy, but you never need a large screen to get the point of these references and, always, the audio is key.

The Bibliography/Videography at the end is
kept very short, but it does give some
references to other work that can add to my
story including my own associated talks and
a few related You Tube talks that you may
find interesting, plus the key video
references in the body of this book.

My warning is that if you skip the videos,
you miss half of what you need to get the
full story. The book is kept short, so you can
read through it fast and go back if you
chose, but if you fail to listen to the
references, you will miss many of the key
points intended.

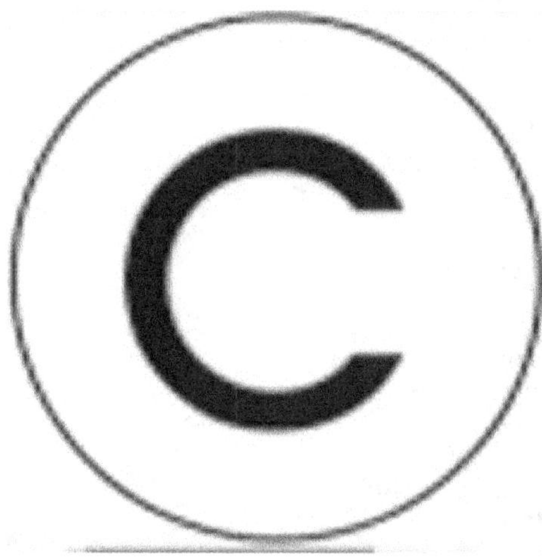

Chapters:

The Dirt

Let's begin with "the real dirt." But first, note that the terms, "dirt" and "earth" can be interposed and are somewhat common in meaning. As it turns out, nearly all of our current health problems can be associated with the condition of "The Dirt." Our soils today are totally lacking in organic minerals and whole nutrients due to modern farming methods. But they also include the addition of oil based fertilizer along with chemicals that contaminate our now totally unrecognizable farmed earth and the previous Earth World in general. Consuming foods grown from these, along with some of our so called medical advancements and other professional recommendations can be associated with most of our health problems today that cause the accelerated aging our real topic herein.

Good organic dirt is either virgin soil or soil that has been re-worked back to allow it to spawn the previous health, wellness, and lifespans of the past well beyond what we commonly encounter today. Thus, it allows antaging to occur on a scale that few now realize or consider possible. We generally have agreed to large scale, high tech, mono-crop farming and living in cites in large, inefficient (and boring) spaces, rather than the efficient, low tech hunter gatherers with small niche multi-crops and natural lighting, as I advocate here, that we once were our common choice. This, results in shortened potential lifespans, which have considerably decreased, despite current reports. This is all documented in stone, as pointed out by Graham Hancock, in referencing the ancient societies below.

As best we can gather, this process actually was under way some 12,860 years ago with the Younger Drias in

ancient Mesopotamia and Gobekli Teki (but likely, many thousands of years prior to that). This period is now recognized by the more adept Historian/ Geologists as the post-flood, or quaternary period, when history was often lost, according to the most profound Archaeologists like Hancock who is interviewed here:
https://www.youtube.com/results?search_query=https%3A%2F%2Fwww.youtube.com%2Fwatch%3Fv%3DIRPGqUdkLdw

Following the Younger Drias, soil depletion became a significant problem as people compensated by living in larger groups. However, more recently, as we introduced artificial, oil based, fertilizers, these problems accelerated with our vast farms supporting dense cities and their millions of people that became possible. Our cities and farms are now considered a desirable asset and certainly not recognized by our experts and planners today as the problem that they have become. Thus, they are endorsed and celebrated by our governments as grand achievements. Yet, these can never

really encompass what is required here
in foods, supplements, etc.

All of the dense supplements pointed
out here generally come from relatively
uninhabited regions (as with Maca),
forests (as with MSM), or our own yards
if we adapt the measures suggested
here.

It you live in a high-rise apartment, you
obviously have no yard, so sourcing
organic dirt and a place to grow things in
is a big issue, but some still try with roof
gardens with some success.

However, if you have a yard (and it need
not be huge) and your garden is
producing healthy products at an
alarming rate using structured water and
good humus soil without harmful oil
based chemicals, you know that you
have re-achieved what nature intended
to nourish your body to its full potential
and with little effort on your part just as
in the past when we hunted, gathered,
and farmed locally in small plots.

Moreover, livestock, raised on this same quality organic dirt that produces fast growing, grasses, when eating them, also reach their natural, most dense nutritive, but now rare potential, when consumed. Here, we are not discussing the commonly termed "free range chickens" and "grass fed cattle." This is about natural grasses and dense organic soils in combination... that is, the wild meadows that greeted arriving settlers when they first set foot in America.

These dense organic, finely ground soils were once created in the Amazon Jungles where they literally farmed humus organic soils there, known as "Terra Preta," as referenced here:
https://video.search.yahoo.com/yhs/search?fr=yhs-pty-pty_email&hsimp=yhs-pty_email&hspart=pty&p=Terra+Parita#id=6&vid=797a4684f57fe8483f2de402748fe2a7&action=view
My own garden has a drain field from my kitchen sink Thus, my plants get "Terra Preta" soil irrigated with highly structured "Living Water." Furthermore, all leftover food goes straight into the mix and is recycled select quality food.

So this soil mix there could be termed "Super Terra Preta."

Read what Howard Garrett, "The Dirt Doctor," one of the few truly expert gardeners today, has to say about this dirty topic, at https://www.dirtdoctor.com Howard has much to add to this story. Also, listen to his weekly talk radio show.

It is comforting that others are teaching the basic organic methods that I have promoted most of my life... that my Grandpa, a brilliant Indiana dirt farmer, passed on to me. This book, however, takes a step back from his wonderful lessons and is really all about relearning what nature had been teaching us for the millions of years prior to these gross practices. So Howard has learned to listen and teach what he is learning himself, directly, and through his listeners. But the number of people that understand what he teaches is still far too small and there is more to add here in concept.

The first person widely heard to report openly on how our soils have been depleted of natural minerals, in recent years, was Dr. Joel Wallach, humorist/ veterinarian. Wallach's initial solution, generally, was to supplement our diets using the colloidal liquid minerals that he marketed. However, below, he expands on this in scope with this recent talk. Here, he begins to lead us toward what I offer as "the next stage" in his lecture:
https://www.youtube.com/watch?v=kihm0QMpYCY

All that Wallach offers helps, but creating a dense, organic dirt is the most basic of health approaches. It provides more than just deficient minerals. Also, as Wallach agrees in his talks, we need vitamins and cofactors to help deliver minerals, but there are also other currently unrecognized vibratory factors in soil. A few cutting edge doctors today discuss the vibratory benefits of walking in bare feet as one aspect of this.

Further, Dr. Dan Nelson, relates how these vibrations affect us here:
https://www.youtube.com/watch?v=7hNW7qxlMzg&t=9s

However, my first key point is with how
organic bioavailable soils are created
as the Dirt Doctor teaches. In doing this,
you avoid harmful chemicals of all kinds
in your garden and yard, especially the
synthetic fertilizers, chemicals, and
weed killers such as "Roundup." This
overall process of awareness and
attitude contribute to getting the sound
and light vibrations back into your life,
along with the huge benefits that they
bring to the table.

Herein, we will revisit the above premise
often. However, we go further as we
address other now forgotten ways that
people have historically, by accident or
by invention, managed to stay well.
Further, I address why a few of us look
so young for our age, while others age
quickly (and, please, this is just not
about genetics or luck, as many would
have you believe today).

The above small scale farming practices,
contributors to slower aging, have
simply been abandoned. Also, modern
medicine and government health

policies have displaced them as the key money makers. With this, they have kept them from being commonly ever practiced today. Unless we reestablish them, we are unlikely to revert back, since applying oil to health solutions always appears more cost effective until you consider the outrageous true costs involved. The quick oil-fix is just not going to carry the day long-term; especially if you want to live in comfort after age fifty or so.

Of course, the common argument today is that aging (and commonly disease) are always genetic in origin. Given this, you, the individual, are left a powerless, irresponsible victim with no real input, control, or understanding. Furthermore, with the above, the only solution can come through high tech manipulation involving chemically based drugs, surgery and radiation that are well beyond your own keen to evaluate. When you accept this premise as true, you yield to the experts and pseudoexperts who in turn yield their power to the government and the

various entities that support it with their huge contributions and advertising budgets. Furthermore, this is contrary to the new science, coined epigenetics, that I reported on in my earlier book, "Beyond Epigenetics." Thus, the totally obvious science of Dr. Bruce Lipton, proves that you are never the "victim" of a powerful gene code that no one can affect. But there is more, as I outline here and Lipton discusses below:
https://www.youtube.com/watch?v=7QxaG9Ng0Is

Nearly everyone today looks at what has occurred in the healthcare and public health sectors as progress and certainly, from some standpoints, it is. Generally, the topics here appear to have downsides or they are hidden from us by politics and even more so by the policies that our bureaucratic government endorses and promotes as healthy advances. The idea here is to take back control of your body and health as Dr. Mercola, discussed later, advocates.

In the long run, some of our old ways may be re-implemented as we wise up

to avoid these quick fixes. First,
reconsider the choices that we are
making that have displaced time
honored practices when vibration was
understood as everything in this
relatively short span of history.

I offer many clues in my first books to
help keep you young. However, the true
fact is that antiaging can never occur if
you are not totally well. So total
wellness and harmonics are really the
key issues here and they run parallel.
First, stay well, nourish your body, and
keep your autoimmune system
unstressed and at full potential. Then,
when applying this vibrational science,
you are only subject to dying from
accidents or wars. With this fact in mind,
it is clear that we should be living many
more years than we currently expect or
we even know possible, as a population
and as Dr. Wallach reports to some
degree in his lecture here.
https://www.youtube.com/watch?v=RYGcHCaDtDM

And his radio show here:
https://www.youtube.com/watch?v=kihm0QMpYC=

Even Colds Age Us

A key factor here is that colds, now considered even the most mild of afflictions, disrupt our harmonics, age us, and move our biological age up at the critical cellular level. You may endure a cold or two every winter as normal, and most endure them as just that. However, not just colds, but all diseases and infections disrupt our harmonics and age us to some degree. Yet colds can be thought of as energy storage attacks at the quantum level as follows:

Colds, literally quantum diseases, reduce your average mitochondrial count per cell (our basic vibratory energy elements) to begin their process. Thus your bioavailable energy, next infection, will be reduced. This is no small price to pay as they shave years off your life in this ongoing procession. Furthermore, there is no mainstream treatment to stop them and all advice is useless for the most part. The key here is to raise your immunity (vibratory potential), so as not to ever catch them

in the first place and there are plenty of
clues here to do that. However, I can be
around people and kids with terrible
colds all day and never catch them.
Thus, the mainstream story is lacking
and incomplete. Below is an explanation
and key intervention till you arrive at this
point yourself:

Oxidation (in iron, is a slow form of
burning, producing heat) ages you, but
without it, your body could not destroy
invaders, DMSO is an powerful oxidant,
so it readily gives up an oxygen
molecule becoming essentially "DMS" or
Dimethyl Sulfone, commonly termed
Methyl Sulfonyl Methane, or MSM, an
equally powerful antioxidant.

Antioxidants are oxygen/free radical
grabbers and MSM is a most powerful
one. So MSM, when ingested, grabs
free radicals and in the process,
becomes DMSO killing various invaders.
Within your body, per the Late Dr. David
Gregg, PhD, it reverts back to MSM as
referenced in my first book. So this is
probably the only true Oxygen Transport

Pair (OTP) that you can ingest by his theory and it is an ongoing transformation. I ingest plenty of MSM daily and an occasional jolt of DMSO. If you are exposed to large crowds in winter, a jolt of DMSO is a good cold/flu preventive, but it is true for all communicable diseases. DMSO is also great topically. When applied to the skin or taken orally, it is tasteless, but hot. Think of that heat as literally burning away (oxidizing) disease and augmenting your autoimmune functions.

Given the obvious power and reported results of these two working in conjunction by so many, the above is the only plausible explanation that makes any sense, but it does require more study. In this process, this OTP preserves mitochondria at the cellular level when combined with geometrically structured "Living Water" even when you have a cold. So the magic is multipart with MSM, DMSO, and structured water with 100% hydration. By the way, the average cellular hydration rate of any reader not taking "Living Water" is about 30%, no matter how much water you consume. As Dan Nelson says, you simply can not raise your hydration rates higher on tap water, no matter how much you ingest, and you tax your kidneys when you drink too much. This is very special stuff, but more on that later.

The accepted mainstream theory behind this oxidation story is that oxygen is the key aging factor. That is, oxygen, to be totally stable, must be a paired molecule with no missing electrons. When free of an electron it is a free radical (lacking one or more electrons). It is thus looking to steal electron(s) from body cells. Again, that kills off mitochondria and ages you. This occurs during a cold and it is why we must teach our bodies to avoid them. Also, review Dan Nelson's commentary on oxygen vs. hydrogen in his talk is a key factor in understanding this at: https://www.youtube.com/user/redelkaudio2

All doctors know that colds can lead to more serious illnesses. It makes total sense and it proves out. While all diseases age us, colds are much more significant contributors than they would appear to be. This, while currently disregarded by science, is actually measurable in the lab. By reducing your immunity, they cause a spiral of microcellular events. In attacking energy reserves at the microcellular level, colds are particularly problematic. They promote free radicals, thus killing off mitochondria and reducing vibratory potential. A particularly bad cold may actually be several recurring attacks, but it is generally seen as one.

What happens with colds and how to avoid them: Physically, colds are not what anyone commonly considers them to be and they are not what is normally described by doctors. By the time the common physical symptoms, termed a "cold," appear, the runny nose, tight throat, etc, the attack is over and the real harm is done. The serious part occurred when your vibratory levels were reduced, your immune system was compromised, and you felt weak. In that process, you suffered a depletion of

mitochondria and resulting massive loss
of vibratory energy..."the real
symptoms." The actual attack is very
similar with what we term as flu, except
with a flu, the aftermath is strong
enough to cause your body to raise your
temperature to kill off the virus.

This energy anomaly was initially set off
when you suffered a loss in UVB
sunlight (which is 70% of your food
source as discussed later), along with
inadequate energy stores. Had you
seen this coming and taken DMSO,
"The world's most powerful oxidant"
along with two micron particle sized
structured "Living Water" and some
vitamin D3, you may have headed this
off when you felt the first tinges of
energy loss. Organic D3 is a necessary
UVB loss preventive in winter when
colds generally occur. Still, you ideally
need to be outside for at least fifteen
minutes at around noon every day or
you risk having even a summer cold.

After the initial attack, some relief can
help by scavenging the created free

radicals. MSM, the king of antioxidants,
works well in conjunction with others
such as organic C,E, and D, etc.

MSM and DMSO should not be ingested
together, since they, in theory, offset
each other. But, again, once one is
ingested, they become the OTP
discussed above. Knowing how many
transfers can occur with one ingestion of
either is the subject of more study.
However, we can generally feel the
effects of both when they are ingested
separately and, especially during a cold.
After a cold, on taking MSM, your
energy levels typically feel replenished,
but the mitochondria remain depleted
unless raised vibrationally as discussed
below.

Finally, the cold fact remains that a
really bad cold considerably reduces
mitochondria counts which can add
years to your cellular age, since
mitochondria are truly where it all
happens. So the bottom line is that you
simply cannot afford to catch colds (or
flu) if you are going to stay off of this

aging spiral discussed here. By avoiding
all illness and cheating the odds in this
crap game of life, we can help slip an
ace up your sleeve with useful clues, if
you are paying attention.

Beyond the above, using vibrational
healing methods, mitochondria counts
can be fully restored. In fact, my friend
Dr. Price routinely raises counts to 2000
avg/cell as a curative to free you of
diseases like Lyme and Malaria as
discussed later. Always, as all true
healers relate, your body heals itself
when given the required biological and
spiritual tools and this is all a part of this.

I absolutely stopped becoming ill, ever,
about ten years ago now. Thus, you too
can actively do things to avoid ever
becoming ill again (colds and flu
included of course), but this is a long-
term process that I go into later herein
as I discuss how we alter vibratory rates
and recognize how it works.

To begin as preparation for the above:
For this to work in the future, the first

key step is that you, in childhood, need
to be "hardened," as I outline below.
From there, stay well from about twenty
years old on to take maximum
advantage of your wellness potential.
Of course, most all of this was unknown
until recently by anyone. I, myself, never
had the benefit of totally understanding
these rather subtle, but now well
understood, scientific factors that I have
arranged into this thesis, suggest to you,
and demonstrate myself.

Still, for me, the most obvious piece
came when colds stopped. At first, I just
considered it good fortune. But now it
has lead to a still unfolding revelation.
So, I am still learning, but its now clear
that you are simply a victim of the
currently prevailing broad mainstream
ignorance commonly masquerading as
medical science that helps sell drugs at
your expense (and theirs too, strangely).

My first book, "It's the Liver Stupid"
comprehensively lays out most of the
supplements and herbs needed in detail
that you must incorporate to make this

total wellness program work for you
personally. However I revisit a few here
that are particularly important beyond
MSM/ DMSO, the key elements,
reported twenty years ago now with the
writing of my first book and further
expanded on here to some degree.

Why Are We So Different?

Disregarding our obvious vibrational
differences that Dr. Bruce Lipton
correctly advances in his talks:

From a purely nutritional aspect, we are
born from mothers that are deficient in
certain minerals and adequate in others
(as one would expect) and this is true in
all animals. Through a pregnancy, as
nature determines, fetuses, grab what
is needed, as required. The fetus is
always given first choice in available
nutrients. Nature is set up to preserve
the species and the fetus is its biological
future, so this is just pure math and logic.

Therefore, the concern here is: "Fetus
Survival" with the mother being a

somewhat expendable means to make it
happen as long as she finally delivers
the baby. This may sound harsh, but
everyone knows it to be a fact. Here,
only nature's intention counts in this
survival story. .
Doctors are always warning about this
indirectly in their drug ads as a part of it,
if you are listening. So whatever the
mother ingests, the fetus gets, first
choice, but it certainly will always grab
any nutrients needed as available. If
there is a deficiency anywhere, the
mother's health will no doubt suffer after
the delivery and this is common. The
bottom line is that the oldest sibling gets
the best nutrient supply and the supply
diminishes with each subsequent
offspring. With this, expect the first born
to be the longest living sibling and many
births are a killer, if there may births, all
for this reason, especially given our poor
diets in general today.

If, for instance, your mother's stores of
sulfur were high enough (rare today),
you may get to age thirty or even forty
with today's inadequate organic sulfur

supplies normally available and with no arthritis or joint problems. A few may develop uncommon eating habits in their upbringing that manage to supply them with enough sulfur to allow them to reach even age fifty without joint failure. Certainly, this is not the norm in the US where our eating habits are atrocious. In fact, this is nearly impossible in all developed countries today.

In an undeveloped country, where sulfur stores might be unusually high, it could be that you are in a locality with low magnesium or some other essential soil nutrient/ vibration that must be supplemented in some manner. Statistics point this out through diseases.

The above, of course, explains why mothers have so many health problems during pregnancy and, commonly today, natural delivery problems, especially in the US. It also explains the sudden dietary/eating urges commonly reported. The obvious fact is that, the mother is going to prematurely age if she becomes very deficient during her term.

But there is a gift: At the second
trimester, as Dan Nelson reports, by
design, the fetus is supplied mineral
vibratory nutrients in a full array,
whether the mother is deficient or not,
for a 21 day period using an encoded
natural genetic program
www.youtube.com/watch?v=7hNW7qxlMzg&t=23s
 (2:18). This program uses Promethium
(Pm, element 61) found in water. Pm, a
fractal, is radioactive with Pm 147 being
the most stable of the group.

The common deficiency story also
explains why doctors recommend
multiple vitamins during pregnancy (as if
that could help). It further explains why
eggs are such good food. If you think
about it, eggs are the embryonic future
of chickens just as fetuses are the future
of people, so nature gives them a leg
up and when you eat them, you get
some of that advantage.

Comment on Multiple Vitamins: In most
all cases, they should be thought of as
drugs and (hint), in fact, most all are
distributed by the major drug companies.
As a result, they are mainly synthetic

substitutes and, in some cases, such as with B vitamins, they actually will cause your body to reject (displace) organic varieties. Thus, multiple vitamins will cause unforeseen problems and deficiencies and thus age you. Read the labels. If they do not list P5P (organic B-6) or Methylcobalamin (organic B-12), throw them away. But the key here, as discussed below, is that you are unique. There is no magic bullet. Buy the organic variety (vibratory form), not the chemical substitute, if you intend to practice what this book teaches and cheat the aging paradigm.

We All Have Arthritis

So never forget that you are an individual with special nutritional needs. No drug company can anticipate them for you and few doctors, or even nutritionists, can ever sort out your dietary needs for you. This is really about careful observation and individual adjustment as needed.

Story: I was at the grocery checkout
counter just a few weeks ago and ran
into my old friend Bob. He asked me
how I was and, I reported fine. He was
limping badly and obviously not so good.
We did not comment on that, because
he already knows what he should be
doing and, for whatever reason, does
not bother. However, the checkout
woman looked at me and said, " He
says that you don't have arthritis?
Everyone has arthritis!"

Bob looked at her and said, "No, Jim
actually does not." I smiled and said
nothing. She obviously did not believe
him. Why would she? She was correct,
everyone over forty today has some
form of joint failure and arthritis just as
Bob does. Arthritis is an essential fact
of life in today's world of chemical
fertilizers, low minerals, and drugs.

Bob illustrates a shining example (at
sixty-five or so) of our normal aging
population. Finally, no one commonly
links arthritis to the heart as a fore
runner to circulatory and heart disease.

However, all are the result of the same
deficiencies and, obviously, they go
hand in hand as I have seen so often. I
can go so far as to predict that once you
have arthritis, heart disease must follow.
So, today, when my friends develop
knee problems, I wait for the other shoe
to drop and it simply does not take that
long to materialize.

Arthritis is a key aging factor in itself, but
is also a prelude to terminal diseases as
noted above. It contributes to why we
look so worn out after seventy or so, as
a population... Furthermore, it is why so
many wheelchairs, walkers, and canes
are sold today, and, for sure, things
have gotten worse. Low sulfur,
magnesium, and organic nutrients result
in: hair loss, soft, slow growing, brittle
nails, white hair, wrinkles, muscle loss.
and other aging factors. But none of this
is totally new as follows:

Even two hundred years ago, long
before our current dominating drug
cartels, if you farmed the same plot for
too long, even using organic fertilizers,

certain minerals were going to become
depleted and your family was going to
become sick... and age. Furthermore,
arthritis predicted, (as the first symptom)
what was coming, and heart disease
would follow, since both are results of
depleted soil vibratory nutrients.
However, joint problems normally lead
the way before the real killers, especially
heart disease and, to a lesser degree,
cancer appeared.

Plants can never just supply back
minerals to themselves and it does not
rain minerals, so your only choice two
hundred years ago was to move on or
become ill as Dr. Wallach cleverly points
out so often on his radio talk shows,
books, and lectures.

Today, with our chemical fertilizers,
weed killers and genetically modified
crops, your food can simply be thought
of as mere pretty plastic representations
of vegetables that help initiate aging and
cause disease just as our artificial
chickens, pigs, and beef cattle do.

Another aspect of all of the above is that our population losses height due to nutrient loss and we consistently gain it back when they are included back in our diet. So test this yourself as I did.

All plants literally eat sunlight and organic soil chemicals as they exist vibrationally, but will dine on what they are fed. They are lazy (or energy efficient if you look at it that way). As we do, they will take what they are given especially when there is little effort required. With this thought in mind, allow me suggest that one good organically healthy stalk of natural asparagus exceeds a normal serving of chemically grown fresh green beans or even supermarket broccoli that mainstream nutritionists consider so very healthy (and are by comparison).

To learn to dowse food quality as Dr. Dan Nelson demonstrates/ discusses on his video (and as I do), watch:
www.youtube.com/watch?v=7hNW7qxIMzg&t=23s (3:36)

I expand on this in earlier books, but you find that you will be hard pressed, in any

supermarket, to find anything of dense
nutritional value, and almost nothing of
https://www.youtube.com/watch?v=7hNW7qxlMzg (1:28)
(2:55)
antiaging value anywhere in this vast
stock of, so called, food, with few noted
exceptions, and as I point out. This
vibrational test is very easily measured
by dowsing and both Dan and Dr. Bruce
Lipton show you how, mostly using
muscle testing methods.

Interestingly, the above includes even
fresh green vegetables and fresh fruit,
not just the canned garbage sold as
food or the dead trash sold as snacks
that predominate our grocery food
shelves.

So mostly, what you eat from a
supermarket will mainly tell your body
that you are starving. This teaches it to
store fat, in the process. In fact, you will
eat more intuitively because it is starving
for nutrients and not getting them, So
you gain weight, in effect, lying to your
own body when you eat this, while
calling it food. With this, you are making
it act like an extremely inefficient

chemical processing plant and thus accelerating the aging process.

To compensate, you may try to wise up and go to the local vegetable stand and buy their fresh stuff, but guess what? They are growing their crops in well defined rows with dead soil, chemicals, and artificial fertilizers. If they were not, the other competing stands would outsell them and their business would not thrive. Look out back from their stand and you will see just how it is done, (and must be done) to compete. Still, this is a better choice to make, and it should get your body to age seventy-five or more. However, it will never do what this book promises is possible.

While the above is true of vegetables, its also true of virtually all farm raised animals. These animals have no choice in their entire lives, but to eat chemically grown corn and to be given drugs to be kept well enough to survive to make it to market (which is in their meat and dairy).

However, for the vegans with the answer: Wild animals, where they exist, are dense, clean sources of nutrition. Still, wild animals often feed on our corn and corn is absolutely the bottom of the barrel when it comes to nutritional energy contributors (even if you consider sugar to be food).

So wild deer feed on corn, since it is an easy meal for them. For them, its like your finding a pile of government printed paper money... you take it without questioning the source, and believe that you have found a gold mine. It may work for you for a very long time, but eventually, it will be worth the same as the paper it is printed on.

Raising Supervegetables

My gardens are not pretty, but are about antiaging. With no pretty straight-tilled rows, I do not turn the soil. In fact, you may see them growing and not even know what you are looking at. There are boarders around my yard, growing plots, places that I pick to grow individual plants, but also places that plants pick to grow well. I commonly move them every few years as sets when they are not so vigorous. Maybe a few strawberry patches can be seen or a blueberry bush if you are paying attention, but all of my garbage is composted to raise the organic level of the soil. Also, as mentioned elsewhere, my kitchen sink drains directly into my garden via a separate 4" perforated drain field of PVC pipe that drains structured "Living Water." As Dan Nelson tells us, its really all about vibrations that they pull from the water, but it is also the vibrations in the water that good organic nutrient dense soils hold.

I am also after diversity... to make it difficult for an invader to launch an attack on of all of my plants at once. I seldom take measures to defend them other than to pick off eggs and worms if they appear.

If you raise strawberries, you know that the third year crop is generally best, and

the plants must be subsequently moved
to bring them back, since they deplete
the soils of their vibrational needs as all
crops do over time and then you must
restore the old plot or move it.

Reluctantly, I push mow my grass to
keep neighbors from reporting me to the
lawn police, but my grass stays happy
and I never bag a single clipping or
fertilize it. Occasionally, I rake some
grass and add the clippings to my
asparagus plants after I allow them to
grow out.

So what do I raise and encourage to
grow in my ugly yard? Certainly berries
and fruits of all kinds, but I love the
antiaging supervegetables However, all
vegetables raised in organic soil beat
anything sold in any store. I list a few of
my own superstars here as follows:

Asparagus:

My favorite garden vegetable occurs in
the spring. It is huge, because, as with
many berries, all you have to do, once it

finds the correct dirt (and it will make its own choice), is harvest the shoots.

Why is asparagus first on my Supervegetables list? One is that it grows extremely fast. In fact, the stalks grow so fast that I can almost see them shoot out of the soil... and as much as two feet in one day after a good rain is common. What this suggests is that the soil is delivering its nutrients as quickly as nature could possibly allow. This, then, is an intense and amazing plant. A key point here is that supervegetables grow fast and that is part of why they are so nourishing. If your soil is great, they are pulling great stuff out of it for you to eat and nourish yourself with.

Asparagus from natural soils is typically two to four times as high in nutrients as that commercially available in stores. So it is a dense source of potassium, when available, (1 gm avg/ serving) and loaded with phytonutrients plus A, B, C, K, E along with other available soil minerals, plus nutrients not even commonly known yet today.

However, a real secret here is in the benefits asparagus carries for your kidneys. Everyone notices the change in urine smell associated with asparagus. But note also that when you eat it every day, this smell basically disappears. Don't expect any huge studies on organic asparagus soon, but if the smell goes away, does it not also make sense that we are also discussing toxins leaving the body?

When you raise asparagus organically, unlike sage government advice, you never wash it and it is generally best eaten raw (with "The Dirt"), or set in boiling water just for a few seconds, to heat it up. However, the fronds never need anything. So if you miss a day harvesting it, just treat the fronds like strawberries or blueberries or other fruit and eat them raw on the spot.

Green Beans:

So the lowly green bean makes my list. Why? Follow me on this... the secret is in the "Dirt," of course. Running to the supermarket will not get you much of anything worth eating, unfortunately.

These are legumes and like all beans can be eaten dried, but when eaten fresh, after they have just shot out (not as fast as asparagus), they deliver a good amount of vitamin K, C, and Manganese (again according to the soils they grow in) and very little, if any, lectin, which can cause digestive issues and weight gain. But organic green beans are packed with nutrients similar to leafy greens, which are not nearly as easy to raise and harvest. They should be picked early before the bean is well formed for their highest nutritional value.

Once these vines start producing, like asparagus, the beans will keep you busy picking them daily. My favorite is pole beans, since they grow, basically, in your face and do not take up a lot of room like grapes. Also, beans are very resistant to pests, blight and similar problems.

On the farm in Indiana, green beans were a family staple. Don't get me wrong, this was in the forties and fifties and already they were being chemically fertilized. But they still tasted great when grandma cooked them all day with bacon grease, lard, and salt; but they were to die for. In those days, I would spend hours in the garden pulling up young carrots and eating them unwashed. No one told me that green beans and young broccoli tasted good raw too. But now I know both are great both raw and in salads.

Today, I find that lightly cooked green beans are good, but they taste nothing like what grandma cooked. Of course, all-day cooked in water means the water carries the same nutrient content as the beans. In those days, that water was simply thrown out. Now, you should know to drink it, because that is where half of the nutrients lie.

Finally, I have only picked two garden supervegs here, but anything grown in organic soils will commonly measure four times the nutrient content of what you buy commercially. I picked these two especially for the reasons I have noted, but also because they grow very fast and they require no upkeep or special consideration.

Maringa Oleifera:

https://www.thespruceeats.com/how-to-prepare-moringa-oleifera-3030161?utm_term=moringa+and+its+health+benefits&utm_content=p1-main-3-title&utm_medium=sem&utm_source=google_s&utm_campaign=adid-5b661afe-cced-49db-87be-b8f186223bc5-0-ab_gsb_ocode-35431&ad=semD&an=google_s&am=broad&q=moringa+and+its+health+benefits&o=35431&gsrc=999&l=sem&askid=5b661afe-cced-49db-87be-b8f186223bc5-0-ab_gsb

Moringa is probably the most nutrient dense vegetable on earth. If not, it is a close second. Nothing commonly marketed today approaches Dried Moringa Leaves for nutrition. Still, there may certainly be something hiding in the dense Amazon Jungle that beats moringa. Also, our next Supervegetable, maca, gives it a run. But below is a rundown on maringa's incredible food value:

Maringa trees are the flowering plants commonly called the Drumstick Tree in native India They grow at an alarming rate... 8-10" a day, plus they are drought resistant. They prefer hot climates, but do OK in temperate zones, seasonally, and can reach 6' to 8' there, dying in winter. Virtually every part of the tree is edible including the roots and bark, but most people stick with the leaves, pods, and seeds. They can be used in soups and provide a nice zest when properly prepared. I commonly eat three level teaspoons of maringa leaves a day and that is about as much as I can handle without causing loose bowels. Yes, maringa can quickly overpower me, so be careful.

https://www.healthline.com/nutrition/6-benefits-of-moringa-oleifera

Maringa oil can be consumed orally, but is used in skin treatments and perfumes and has been around for thousands of years. Please note: Again, this is extremely powerful stuff, but you absolutely need it in any comprehensive diet.

So from here, we move into the superfoods that you normally buy, with minor exceptions:

Cacao:

This is raw coco... the stuff that, combined with sugar, becomes the dark chocolate that doctors commonly recommend. Cacao commonly has so much organic magnesium in it that you can easily deliver all of this critical, essential mineral that you need daily, with no downside, and it tastes good all alone or mixed with such things as Whey, Maringa, and Maca with a little Cream or Goat Milk, as I do and it can be a full meal. If your muscles tend to cramp, take more, but a heaping teaspoon, two to three times a day, should keep them nice and relaxed.

The common suggestion that chocolate is good for you is true... but raw. Try eating raw, chocolate once, without the sugar, and you will see why Cacao is the right answer for this one. Raw

Cacao tastes really good when used alone or in the above mix. Either way, you will be getting the single most heart disease preventive that you could be ingesting that few get enough of today.

Maca:

This stuff will absolutely boost energy levels beyond belief:

For men: https://www.reference.com/health/benefits-maca-root-men-6c45369ac6e48e5c?aq=health%20benefits%20of%20maca%20root

For women: https://www.reference.com/health/benefits-maca-root-women-6f7181d1e693eb3b?aq=health+benefits+of+maca+root&qo=cdpArticles\

My experience is that the benefits of Maca Root, in all of its colors, are actually understated. This is a kick-ass vegetable in every way. It will raise your energy levels and hold them there without your even being aware of its action. Like maringa, it has been around for thousands of years and I just cannot get enough of it, ever, but three heaping teaspoons a day is a start.

The more I take, the better everything seems to work and I take plenty in all colors... but at least three heaping teaspoons daily keeps me on the ball. I wonder what my energy levels would be if like if I took a cup a day or more, could I stand it... could they? My tennis game seems to always improve when I take more. Plus, as reported, the whispering is true. Generally, things that have a reputation for raising libido have overall benefits. Moreover, it seems to raise my mental factors along the way, so If you are pulling an all-nighter in college, you want a good supply of maca on hand to get you through the night and finals.

Coconuts:

Coconuts are indeed supermarket supervegetables despite the report that follows. They can, of course, be consumed in many forms and all forms are very nourishing. One of the things that saves them is that they do not need oil based fertilizers to grow and they are

prolific. So they grow just about
anywhere without fertilizers. That alone
makes them special.

So when you buy a coconut in the
supermarket (of all places) you are
actually getting an organic product that
is totally life sustaining (hard to believe!).
Always read the labels, but coconut oil
will last a long time without chemical
additives and it will sustain high heat
without giving up its nutrients.
Everything considered, Coconut Oil is
likely the best cooking oil on earth (if
you must cook with an oil) and
seasoned with vinegar it makes a great
salad dressing.

Interestingly, coconut milk is as
powerful as structured "Living Water" or
Dan Nelson's "Wayback." That is, it is
100% hydrating. Moreover, since it is
full of nutrients that you are not likely to
encounter anywhere else, it has a huge
plus side. So coconut milk is magic stuff
in itself.

The Downside of Coconuts:

The Mayo Clinic (ref. below) tells us there have a been a few "small studies" that look closer at the effectiveness of using coconut oil, which they say is high in calories and saturated fat in shedding pounds. More on shedding pounds later, but keep in mind that this could also mean that there have not been any useful studies proving how weight loss really occurs. Further, given my own analysis, I suggest, it means that previous studies regarding weight loss are simply bogus. High calories and fat are, as I report below, simply not the base problem regarding weight loss and several experts agree here:
https://www.youtube.com/watch?v=MPPkMhDfDK0

Furthermore, when you look at our population today, what we are being told about weight loss is obviously not accurate. Virtually all current science disregards the now proven fact that your body is a quantum machine. With that, all common assumptions and studies are likely subjective and incorrect. This

means that we have a lot of text books
that constitute useless shelfware.

Certainly, no one wants to be
overweight and we are all trying to be
slim and beautiful, but none of this is
obviously working at all and this is
mainly a fairly recent problem. Look at
the wall paintings in Egypt... fat people?

Here you are getting the word on foods
that you can produce yourself in a small
yard and on a small budget. Coconuts
and these others are inexpensive. With
these, when you avoid the sugar and
carbs that are being pushed on you to
addict you and if you follow the circles
and arrows here, you will absolutely lose
weight. More on that later, but counting
calories does not work and these
superfoods are something that will help
keep you trim.

Furthermore, anyone who still believes
that saturated fat is a dietary problem is
still stuck in the "statinville" drug culture
where most of the clueless drug

vampires live today. When will we free our society of them?

I further discuss weight gain and loss in detail later. But the fact is that, today, our understanding of how this amazing quantum body works is seldom close to what we are being told. In fact, if you are an expert and swear that you understand how the vibrations that sustain us get into the mitochondria, no matter how many doctorates you hold, I maintain that you are clueless.

I further suggest here that what is really happening is simply beyond what any mind can comprehend. To prove this to yourself, start with what is modeled with the three methylation cycles and consider that what they are saying does not even suggest how these very complex energy transfers occur. This transport system is truly rocket science times a trillion... for the 7 trillion cells.

https://www.usatoday.com/story/news/nation-now/2017/06/16/coconut-oil-isnt-healthy-its-never-been-healthy/402719001/

Consider that if no one really knows the true workings of the energy transport system, no amount of education can teach it. That is where we are with these human bodies at the Quantum Level that we occupy and I suggest that likely, we will never fully understand how these esoteric transfers occur. However, the best explanation is just to say that it is vibrational, just as sound vibrates a tuning fork, and that is likely as much as we can mentally grasp. But I did try to cover this with deep, thought provoking references in my last book.
"Crystal Clear Vibrations"
http://rewards-2017.com/amz/index3.php?domain=www.amazon.fr

Keep in mind that these people do not get that structured water and magnetism are vibrations and include sound which emits light as now commonly accepted.

Government Health

Today, our public health concerns end up being global warming, providing inoculations for all children, and finally having enough clean water and health

care facilities. Interestingly, while none
of these make my list, I discuss them in
earlier books in detail. The "Dirt" here is
that you are given solutions to problems
that you can mostly affect positively if
you take the time and effort yourself,
but we are moving mountains, so this
book is a catwalk, not a cakewalk. So
the "Dirt" is about local, not
monumental solutions.

I have come to believe that if a
Government Agency tells you something
related to diet, if you do the opposite,
you will likely be making the wise choice.
Certainly, you will never likely hear a
government agent say that our dirt is
depleted of organics or how our
chlorinated city water will eventually
make you sick. Yet these are basic
premises in this and my earlier books.
Officials want you quiet and happy as
you march in lockstep to an early grave
and lessen their conceived
overpopulation problem, but did they
notice that they too are in step?

Supplementation

So the bottom line here, if you are interested in living beyond eighty with any degree of functionality and richness in your life, is to seek out the supplements that count... to put the vitality back that you are missing from the foods that you were designed to eat eons ago.

In fact, once you understand how this all works, you discover that you hardly need any food at all. It seems that as hunter gatherers, we simply were not that good at getting anything like the amount of food that people typically consume today. Still, when they got food in the distant past, the density and quality was high. My own observation today is that 1/4 pound of dense meat and vegetables grown from organically dense dirt per day will sustain you, but more on that later.

So the key in all of this is more about nutrient density and not quantity. But the real key is the nutrient density of the dirt that the plants grow in. More globally, if the animals that feed on them consume them in that food chain and little else, they will pass on the density.

However, importantly for us, there are still supplements (Foods) today, that live in the Amazon and mountains of Peru that are incredibly dense. Eight level teaspoons a day of these (like Maca and Maringa) will sustain you and even put weight on you, if you fail to get the exercise and keep your metabolism up. This I discuss and prove later here with careful personal observations.

So back to those childhood diseases that help your body learn who you are so it can avoid later confrontations: Let's begin with some "Dirt" that many professionals report occasionally, but most seldom discuss, since they refute common practice today:

Water

No discussion of nutrition, food, or dirt is complete without some reference to water. Water, a harmonic crystalline substance itself, is the basis for all life and, interestingly, within our body, it fills our Pineal Gland, along with harmonic solid crystals. With these, it allows us to dream, create, and transcend our current functional levels beyond all that most understand. So with this, the higher the structural potential that the water itself carries, the greater its effect and the effects and the more spiritually transforming it is. When the water is charged as this "Living Water" is, you can expect huge health benefits, but especially spiritual benefits as your pineal gland initiates those harmonic crystals as you dream.

Our two micron "Living Water," created by pouring water through an encoded proprietary Crystal/ Fractal set, raises your the pineal gland's ability several thousand times its current level. This means that the water alone is spiritually transforming without doing anything else.

I have reported on this water in detail and shown how Plants have grown at 3x normal rates. Commercial growers report similar results. This is a profound technology that can multiply world food production levels and improve even biologically raised superfoods well beyond current levels.

https://www.youtube.com/watch?v=73o0 (30:0) IBUsfr0

So plants respond similar to people in ways that we do not understand. With your body, your pineal, a tuning fork, is vibrating these crystals and in the process, storing new information that your mind and heart never previously had access to.

If you are not ready spiritually, this commonly translates to dreams, so as not to overly disturb you. From here, your mind grabs what it can deal with till it is ready to process the complete story and release it to you in total awareness. This process could take hours or lifetimes to complete according to your level on the spiritual ladder of life, but you will eventually get it all at some point no matter where you happen to be spiritually at the moment.

Healthy Parasites

Unless you are exposed to parasites at a young age, as many have come to realize, your body simply fails to recognize and defeat them as you grow older. That is, our autoimmune system may fail to recognize the problem and attacks itself or the wrong thing. This is true of parasites as well as childhood diseases that we are now inoculated against (inoculations, in some cases, required by law). So we are simply too clean and too removed in this process of childhood adjustments. These dirty aspects always were there in the past and even necessary, but they were certainly never sought out and were always considered an annoyance

The other side of the coin is that when these never come into play, because our bodies are inexperienced, the immune system attacks things that are not problems... referred to today as autoimmune diseases. While around previously, they are now common due our new found cleanliness.

As a result, we have a generally weak society that is ill equipped and unable to cope with our current biological world in the ways that previous generations did. Even more, our biological world has, of course, become more nasty with our addition of oil based chemicals and radioactive fallout, so we require higher immunity levels than ever before. Furthermore, our medicine attempts to make up for our weakness with drugs. This mostly exacerbates our problems rather than to ameliorate or resolve them.

Today, nearly all of the population is in some way allergic to something. Just ask anyone under age 60. But be prepared, as they give you a rundown on their list of problems that in a group of sixty somethings is often the main topic today (along with joint issues). While there is no proof, I suggest that this was not generally the case three hundred years ago, if you compare their correspondence to ours today. Certainly, once past childhood, they were a very hardy group of people then with very few allergies.

Below we consider all forms of parasites from bacteria to protozoan. Additionally, we address the balancing act that a healthy body must go through to maintain wellness and why so few today know the importance of good dirt as opposed to modern day toxins in helping to reject the harmful parasites that feed on our weaknesses.

In all of this, the two most harmful parasites existing in the world today, the ones that kill the most people, are the seldom discussed Malaria and Lyme Disease. While a very few of us already have natural defenses against them, most of us, with the proper nutrients can develop them as I discuss here. Specifically: Lyme disease, especially in the US, and Malaria, in Africa, are in this category. Finally, I cover ways to avoid them and what can be done once you contract them if you never develop these defenses.

But before that, let's begin with some of the darker parasites in terms of what can sometimes kill people, but can also heal them, when under the control of a fully stimulated autoimmune system as explained:

Nematodes (Round Worms)

Many varieties of roundworms can cause problems in humans and plants. They are very simple un-segmented worms of the Nematoda Phyla and do not increase in number from larval form to adult worms. These grow larger through an increase in cell size not by adding more cells as we do. There are over 89,000 identified species today and possibly one million or more that have yet to be identified. Of those, 15,000 have been identified as problematic and some sixty are known to cause terrible problems in humans today. A few are life threatening and they can cause such things as River Blindness in Africa, a disease that is even difficult to discuss, let alone see its results.
https://www.youtube.com/watch?v=QpVF9EnZFn

Dropping back several notches though, the most common and pervasive nematodes are hookworms and whipworms which commonly infect children in developing countries, mostly in rural areas, today. But interestingly, hookworms were especially common with farm kids here in the US just fifty years ago and were almost universally carried by them. However, they were generally asymptomatic, long term. Commonly, they nearly universally caused a mild anal itching among kids who grew up on farms. People my age, generally, recall them as kids before they went to sleep at night, but no one seemed worried or cared. Rarely, they caused anemia, colitis, diarrhea, and with extreme infections, rectal prolapse.

As nasty as these worms sound, their presence and the "dirt" that they came from, commonly horse and cow manure, actually helped us to avoid the suffering from the common allergies so prevalent in society today as we matured.

It is now generally understood today that these worms activated our auto-immune systems as we matured with their "Dirt." So Pin Worms may have been an uncomfortable necessity for a few years, but they were an integral part of humanity for many thousands, likely millions, of years that helped teach our bodies, a degree of awareness they is totally uncommon today, just as childhood diseases did. Indeed, our bodies learn from our actions and exposures in ways that we as a society ignore today for the most part.

On reaching our teen-age years, our systems were wise enough to create the antibodies, bacteria, etc. necessary to rid themselves of these round worms, so these infections could not survive long. Also, our heath levels by then were developed enough, given the quality of food consumed in that era, that they never became more than mild infections.

Typically, round worms numbered less than 100 worms in a healthy child even at their highest levels. So the bottom

line is that they were beneficial in that
they taught our autoimmune systems
how to be activated and helped keep us
strong for our remaining lives. Today,
with our clean environments, these
parasites, as well as childhood diseases,
are both rare in the US.

As a result, nearly everyone under the
age of fifty today, universally, suffers
from allergies of all types and, obviously,
some of these make their lives
unbearable. Therefore, we employ
Immunologists, expertly trained doctors,
who do nothing but treat people in these
areas with a long list of drugs that have
been developed to control them (along
with their harmful associated side
effects), when used in the treatment.

While it is unlikely that any doctor today
will introduce pin worms into a child's
system to keep their immune systems
perked up, the truth is that our society is
just too clean (and most any
immunologists will agree). Yet, only
occasionally is this discussed.

So these nematodes (and the dirt
associated) served a universal function,
just as did childhood diseases like
chickenpox and mumps once did in my
era, since had already been inoculated
against small pox. But now, it is
considered essential that children be
inoculated prior to school for all of them
and often well before their immune
systems have developed to any degree
to resist the response to these
inoculations.

Today, my good friend, Dr. Richard S.
Price has determined that he can readily
eliminate Nematodes just as he does
most parasites, and quickly, through the
vibrational healing methods that he has
developed.

Given the above, my question here is:
Should we employ nematodes as a form
of inoculation similar to the Salk vaccine,
but against autoimmune dysfunction? In
many autoimmune diseases, if done, we
could likely get rid of allergies and
eliminate autoimmune diseases along
the way. Thus eliminating such diseases

as MS, RA, Lupus, ITP, Chrone's, and others. Treatment today for these is commonly cordical steroids, which actively reduce our immune system response (for obvious reasons). How much sense does this make to you?

The above may sound a bit radical, but consider that we were introducing live polio viruses until only recently into all children with the Salk Vaccine. No one in the US commonly contracts polio today, but virtually everyone in the US has some form of allergy at some time in their lives, and the problem is rampant in younger people today along with the above list of autoimmune conditions. Also, autoimmune diseases are now thought to be an outcome of all of this, since they were far less known prior to the above.

So this was one form of nematodes that did some good with our older crowd that no longer help our population. Below is another form that was in no way a problem for people, ever, but these are

very helpful in reducing plant problems
naturally as follows:

Beneficial Nematodes

These were once a common part of the
biology of all open areas and since
some birds commonly use mud to build
nests, they were likely spread as a part
of their healthy habitat. However, many
of the chemicals sprayed on or near
crops today have killed them off to a
great degree and they need your
assistance to again proliferate.

Barn Swallows are one example of a
species that builds nests of mud & sticks
that once had no such protective cover
to keep them out the rain. With no nest
moisture, these nematodes cannot exist
and they are not transferred so much as
they once were, since their nests are
generally covered by roofs.

There are several varieties of these
beneficial nematodes available from
distributors including HB and SF
varieties that can be applied to your

lawn to combat fleas, larval worms, ticks, wasps, various plant infections, termites, mosquitoes, harmful nematodes, tarantulas, spiders, chiggers, and about any other vermin that one could imagine smaller than a mouse. In fact, for instance, chiggers, which were not very common in our East Coast area have begun to appear. This is also likely because these nematodes have been killed off by current farming chemicals and practices.

The cost of a treatment runs between $20 and $60 according to the area treated and, once done, they can become a permanent part of your soil. So this could be one way to ward off Lyme disease in the US and Malaria in Africa without any harmful spraying or chemical treatment.

There are several methods of application, but most employ the mixing of the Nematodes into water and spreading them by spraying them on the soil in the evening, preferably just before

a rain. Watering them after application
helps also. Please watch:
Brad the bug man who sells Nematodes
on sponges:
https://www.youtube.com/watch?v=sXPJJx_U4E0
https://www.youtube.com/watch?v=sXPJJx_U4E0
Controlling various larva with
Nematodes:
https://www.youtube.com/watch?v=5iE-gzC2dy8
Watch how effective these worms are
against the black vine beetle... amazing
pictures:
https://www.youtube.com/watch?v=jM4kZsQntxU
Professional greenhouses using
nematodes.
https://www.youtube.com/watch?v=Y67yhIIQdLU

While adding Nematodes, Ladybugs
are another form of beneficial and
natural biology that should be
encouraged: Ladybugs do not benefit
your health directly, but you want them
to be in your yard and garden along with
the nematodes and below is a great
summary of how to encourage them in
your yard along with the nematodes:
https://www.youtube.com/watch?v=exjuH-Wpc6Q

So encourage ladybugs (beetles) in your
yard. The above lets you into how their

larva and adult stages help to keep
down the problem insects in your
garden and avoid chemicals. So avoid
the chemicals that others use that help
poison their lawns and their bodies in
the process.

In my own garden: All of the boarders
and trees act in some way to produce
edible fruits and vegetables today.
Some of the trees serve as arbors for
grapes. Blueberries, strawberries, and
broccoli and lettuce make nice border
crops, but I also raise a vegetable
garden for food crops.

Antibiotics

Interestingly, as previously reported,
nematodes are known to cause a mild
anemia among kids. My doctor at age
five decided that I was indeed anemic
and attempted to give me penicillin.
Why? No one seemed to know then and
my mother was not too happy that her
diagnosis or treatment that she
determined required a penicillin shot per
week.

However, at age 3, I especially avoided
her treatment whenever possible and
hid behind our couch when she came to
our house with her needle to treat my
condition. We fortunately moved and
the anemia, if it ever existed at all,
subsided on its own, along with those
pin worms that we all had.

Even more interestingly, today,
allergies are also one of the reported
possible side effects of penicillin. In the
forties, penicillin was the newly
discovered, misunderstood miracle drug
of that era. So today, given the
popularity of penicillin, which most
everyone agrees was greatly overused,
we have replaced it with a hundred new
antibiotics per the list below with known
side effects and these side effects are
even less understood.:
https://en.wikipedia.org/wiki/List_of_antibiotics

These, most also agree, are overused
and, as a result, will end up being no
better than penicillin as they produce
stronger, more efficient, and more

powerful bacteria that nothing can cope with in our hospitals.

Avoid Parasitic Diseases

Obviously, one way to avoid malaria entirely is to avoid mosquitoes by spreading nematodes per the above and as recommended by Howard Garrett, "The Dirt Doctor" on his radio show. However, in tropical climates, they experience a long, warm, rainy season and people are crowded, so possibly nematodes are not the best solution there.

A second way to nip this problem in the bud, as I have reported in the past is to take MSM/LW *MSM with structured "Living Water"). over a long period. Then, as I have experienced, you are no longer bitten by mosquitoes at all. Thus your body chemistry simply changes. Mosquitoes still fly near and buzz you, because you are warm, but they simply never land on you and never bite. So this treatment, when taken over a long period is obviously the most direct way

of combating malaria, making both
Malaria and Lyme diseases (discussed
below), essentially become non-
diseases entirely. This alone, if done
worldwide, could likely eliminate
700,000 deaths a year.

Beyond mosquitoes, with MSM/LW,
strangely, as I have reported, your
blood chemistry actually changes so
drastically that bee, wasp, and yellow
jacket stings no longer cause any
swelling or itching.

Moreover, since the toxin in stinging
insects is very similar to those of
poisonous snakes, it is reasonable to
assume (as a few have reported on You
Tube also) that these will not affect you
either.

While these reports may be true, I do
not plan to voluntarily test this one on
myself. In fact, I never have tested any
of these on purpose. I simply
discovered them by mistake.
Nevertheless, when wasps do sting me
today, there is no toxic effect and no

swelling, but mosquitoes, along with this, have stopped biting me altogether. Never in human history is there evidence that the above was a factor in malaria, but others today have confirmed all of this and I now can report, that it is true. Still, it was all an unexpected outcome.

In fact, a few report that mosquitoes never naturally bit them and I know this also to be true. However, in my case, I was obviously extremely attractive to mosquitoes just a few years ago and their bites ten years ago caused huge welts, so this is absolutely not my imagination.

Also, as a child, chiggers seemed to have loved digging into my skin on the farm in Indiana and, in those years, I was always pulling out embedded ticks because I loved the woods. So this phenomenon, for me, is all a relatively recent side effect from my taking high levels of MSM over a long period and a few report them to me who have followed this MSM program.

Malaria:

Lets begin with malaria as a disease: There are five (or more, according to how you classify them) parasites delivered by mosquitoes (primarily Anopheles). The symptoms of each varies, but they all, at some point, attack the red blood cells and cause seriously high fever and uncontrollable shaking that literally reaches into the bones of the host. Since each variety attacks in different ways, the discussion here will mostly address the Ovale. However, they are all protozoan parasites, once in the body, and they are all classified as Plasmodium, since they all attack red blood plasma:

Ovale: This variety is endemic to West Africa and is often considered less harmful than the others. However, the reason may be that it is simply slower acting. Long term, it may be the most destructive of all.

To begin, any plasmodiam species can lie dormant (erythrocytic stage) in the system for months before it breaks out into the blood. When it attacks, the initial attack may only last for a day or two, then it goes back into what is considered this dormant phase. Before that, it may attack again within a short period and kill the victim because they have exhausted them.

Now lets, first off, point out that any parasite that kills its host is not successful, since it dies with them. So any good parasite does not kill... at least quickly. Long term, this Ovale, with its complications is a different story as follows:

What occurs after the initial infection(s) is that the plasmodium invades one or more vital organs. Commonly, the liver first, then it actively moves to the kidney's, the spleen, and any vital organ is fair game (except the heart). But in this stage, Ovale is mostly asymptomatic and the host believes that they are well. They can feel just fine

until an organ actually begins to fail,
then the person may believe that they
have, for instance, a kidney infection,
and it goes on from there.

So when the person's infected organ(s)
begin to fail, doctors, even those
regionally familiar with the parasite,
commonly are unaware of the actual
cause and commonly assume it to be
bacterial. Assuming that it is bacterial,
they employ a broad spectrum antibiotic.

Not only is an antibiotic useless against
a plasmodium parasite, any antibiotic
use reduces the immune system's ability
to control the problem by killing bacteria.
So the result is that the host loses some
ability to hold off the parasite as they
multiply. Thus, the host becomes
weaker and more ill as a result. This
sequence, when repeated over time,
can easily result in the failure of the
organ and likely an infection of the other
kidney (or organs). So if it was one
kidney, now it is both. Thus, dialysis
could be one outcome and eventually
death as other organs are invaded.

So the assumed cause, the bacteria, was never a problem. The good gut bacteria never had a chance. Further, the prognosis is poor once this chain of events occurs. Never is an antibacterial treatment a benefit once the treatment is completed, as outlined previously.

My limited experience with malaria, is that DMSO will kill the parasite in its erythrocytic phase in the kidney in a less than an hour. But vibrational healing will cause the parasite to leave the host totally in a matter of minutes and that kills nothing. Parasites are designed to survive just as the host is. With vibrational healing, everyone wins and this is the ideal solution for all parasites including protozoan or bacterial as you will see and as we move into this softer form of medicine of the future.

So while DMSO alone is apparently very effective against malaria, the ideal is to allow the parasite to continue to live, but to move it to a different vibrational realm.

The key here is that no matter how
much we may hate malaria, it deserves
to live. With vibrational healing, the
protozoan is slipped into a different
spiritual realm or "zone" where they do
not affect people negatively, so all are
happy. The expression is that we just,
"Want them to go away, but not to go
away mad."

So what would happen if we employed
DMSO as a common treatment for
Ovale malaria? Well, likely, it could kill
off malaria in Ghana, but there are
karmic implications in killing anything,
despite all current opinion. This is just
not the way to deal with life. The use of
antibiotics or any of today's common
treatments carries those same
implications to some degree. Swatting
flies does too, but few avoid doing of it,
even me.

This is no different. All healing, done
well, is best done at the vibrational level
where there are no repercussions. We
may not consider smaller forms of life as
life, but there is always a better method

of disease and parasite control.
Correctly viewed, even the worst
parasites are beneficial in some way.

This explains all of the other forms of
malaria if you are interested:
https://www.youtube.com/watch?v=2O3YrdUZQ5U
Malaria larvae live in the Erythrocytic
phase, where they vary from 72 hours
with Plasmodium Falciparum to infinite.
Herein, I suggest that despite this, the
others exhibit far worse initial symptoms.
But long term, Ovale is likely the worst
variety, because it stays in the
Erythroytic phase the longest. In this
phase, they attack vital organs and can
kill as "complicated malaria," as noted
above. Here it is generally not even
recognized as malaria by most doctors,
even in areas of high malaria infections.

Chemoprophylactic treatments, as we
hear, cause problems that keep them
from working if you take them after
contracting malaria. Why? Because the
parasites become normalized just as
with antibacterial treatments against
bacteria. So, despite the "feel good"
advice spread by the Bill Gates crowd,

there is no direct cure for malaria in mainstream drugs today, no matter how much money is thrown at it.

Most people believe that when they are going to travel to Africa, they can be inoculated against malaria. That is simply a feel-good approach for westerners. If you are white skinned and stay long, you have a nearly a 100% chance of contracting malaria if bitten by a single carrier.

If you contract malaria, you can drink quinine water in the active events to help mitigate it. However, you are likely to die of organ failure of Ovule, once contracted, somewhere down the road in life. Then, nothing can be done other than to treat symptoms, using current medicine, despite reports to the contrary. Just hope that you are not treated with antibiotics!

In the video below, I explain dowsing and discuss healing and why we become ill, ever here:
https://www.youtube.com/watch?v=0U7pI14L3sU

"Cancer & Disease Prevention Using Fractals." So will you avoid malaria totally if your level of health is high enough? Theoretically, yes, but herein I give you ways to totally avoid all parasitic diseases and some ancillary help that few know. This was only a few years after I became disease free, so I was only becoming aware of the possibilities at this point. However, it is clear now that with this could completely eliminate all parasitic disease with no medical intervention or disease countermeasures.

Lyme Disease

So we have a way to avoid ticks in your yard using nematodes and that is helpful. I have yet to definitely prove that MSM stops ticks from ever digging their heads into my skin, even though I never have had a tick bite me in ten years . But I still commonly go into infested areas today. Allowing a tick to dig in is just not a test that I prefer to conduct, like poisonous snake bites, though. I hate these critters and find them obnoxious.

The question is, if they never crawl on
me, would they ever dig in if they did?
Of course they could, but I am happy
enough avoiding them and never being
bitten. So I am not going to test this
hypothesis even though it appears true.
Furthermore, I am not about to subject
myself to a rattlesnake or cobra bite for
science. By the way chiggers, no longer
like my taste either, so far, and they are
related mites. Again, chiggers ate me
up as a kid when I helped pick wild
blackberries with my family.

Knowing all of the above, in my opinion,
you really have no business contracting
Lyme disease. However, for those who
have not gone through the five to ten
years or so required to build up the
immunity using MSM: Dr. Price can
fairly easily put an end to Lyme Disease
and Malaria vibrationally and I have
witnessed it. If you have contracted
either, all is not lost and he teaches his
skills to others, so it could become
common.

Lyme is commonly initially treated with
massive antibiotics. The result is that it
drives them deeper and causes the
survivors to morph into resistant
varieties. Thus, you think you are well,
but ten or twenty years later, expect bad
things to happen. In this way, it shares a
lot with malaria. When you get a second
outbreak, like malaria, prospects are
not too encouraging. With a third
outbreak, there is almost no chance of
survival, long term.

Still the best treatment for Lyme and
Malaria is to have Ticks and Mosquitoes
avoid you entirely by making yourself
unattractive to them as I have.

Ringworm

I picked ringworm of the foot or athletes
foot ringworm here, because most of us
have, at some point, contracted it.
However, this could be any one of
several common afflictions that are not
in any way life threatening, but can
cause itching problems and outbreaks
even for those on this MSM protocol:

Ringworm is not a worm at all, but a
fungus. I address it here because it is
so prevalent. I still get it occasionally
and little is known about it in medicine
today.

Also, we were warned about it starting in
grade school and seldom given the
correct facts. So I still have occasional
outbreaks for no apparent reason and
never am I around others afflicted with it,
which makes no sense, given what we
are told.

The cause of Ringworm is obviously not
well understood, since it is commonly
described as dampness related fungus
that is contracted from others in
showers, etc. This is just not the case
as the woman in the video below reports.
How does this make any sense when
she only had it on her chest, neck and
face and not between her toes or on her
feet? Agreed, these are uncommon
locations, but I recall clearly having had
it on my hands in 6th grade, where it
went away on its own:
https://www.youtube.com/watch?v=XIB5kHobIal

Some organic ringworm cures she
suggested are Garlic, Tea Tree Oil,
Eucalyptus, Coconut Oil, but mix them
with DMSO (the oxidative state of MSM)
and one application of this is often good
enough to initiate a cure.

My cure, and it is really fast, is to break
the raised puss nodes with a needle and
apply the 100% DMSO mix liberally. It
is immediate and the itching stops with
no further spread, generally.
No matter what the problem, the key
here is that when you use even a
commercial over-the-counter cure or
the above mixed with DMSO, a liquid
(there are DMSO cream preparations
available), you are cured. With DMSO,
the effectiveness and cure time is
increased many fold and this is true for
similar problems using DMSO. If there
was ever a magical general cure and
delivery system, DMSO qualifies.

Our Bodies are Listening
Short Term Lessons

We are intelligent beings (to varying degrees), but most are not aware that we are constantly training our quantum bodies in this process of life and gaining in intelligence. So here we discuss how this process works and how it is key to wellness and longevity.

Our bodies are comprised of some 70 Trillion cells (according to how you figure) and these cells are basically specialized groups. Listen to:
https://www.youtube.com/watch?v=-2yvmp7yn_l

Each body cell is a totally aware individual, like a specialized protozoan species, but also in this survival process it knows everything that is going on with the rest of them (your body cells) as self protection. Thus, your cells are listening and they feel your overall vibrations. Furthermore, you converse with them on various levels. With this, your liver certainly knows about your heart, but to a degree, so does your skin know about your eyes.   The key here is that you are not an isolated mind, as we are taught today. We, as individuals, are a part of a deep overall and ongoing inner conversation.

Beyond all of that, what you do in your physical life gives your cells some idea of how to plan. You may not believe that this is possible, but this feedback has implications on how fast you age and your total wellness. So, be aware that nothing occurs in this orchestration in a vacuum.

Therefore, your organs need to be fed in specialized ways so that they can think clearly and plan ahead and they absolutely do. Furthermore, when you stress an organ by depriving it of its specialized fuel (the proper nutrients/ vibrations), it will be affected adversely and it will take steps to compensate. Too much stress and it may become inflamed, thus, a target for bacteria and parasites, or worse, it may totally fail. Examples of the most serious of these

are heart an liver failure. This is all an
extension of what Dr. Lipton teaches in
his interview above and what Dan
Nelson tells us.

Keep in mind that most of what we feed
our cells today has no resemblance to
what nature set up for our cells to live on.
That is, the organic foods are missing.
These were meant to be raised under
quantum conditions with a full
complement of specialized vibratory
nutrients that are unaltered by both
chemicals and men's ideas. To remain
totally well and thus antiage, you first
need both a great attitude and then the
correct vibratory foods to accomplish
these lofty goals.

Interestingly, our are men of science
today actually believe that they can
improve on what nature adjusted your
cells to live on and hear over these
millions of years. This scientific
conviction may indeed speed up our
food production process and make
money for their marketers. However,
this attitude certainly cannot in any way

improve your health outcomes and
goals, so your cells will certainly feel the
brunt of this failing experiment that I am
suggesting here you can avoid with
some effort.

Your job, then, is to find less altered
supplements and foods that are more
close to what your cells and organs look
for if you ever want to age beyond your
currently allocated 80 years with any
degree of wellness. This search, as you
can see, is quantum science and literally
it is completely the opposite of rocket
science. Instead of explosively forcing a
projectile through space, our method is
to open up a spiritual time window, then
to allow yourself to be drawn through
time gracefully in full awareness.
Most of the animal and plant foods that
you eat have undergone very similar
stresses to our human population given
the chemicals fed them. That is, they
eat those same refined chemicals
(mainly based on oil), that are putting
our own cells at risk... but also, putting
our plants and livestock cells at risk in
this circle of life that is a continuum. We

are forcing life on today almost as if we are squeezing it through a narrow opening that can never accommodate it.

In the most simple terms, what the continuum needs is just good dirt. That is, inorganic and oil based chemicals are just not what your cells need and there are no shortcuts that science can create. Therefore, even if you are keeping in touch with them spiritually, your cells deprived of these whole earth minerals, must break. They simply do not fit. For this reason, our synthetic current conversation starts failing at around 75-80 years.

However, unfortunately at 80, you are a spiritual child and this is the point where we are just coming out of this cloud. At 80-85 years, you are spiritually set up to begin the greater journey... to set the world on its ear. The key here is that we finally are able to work with both sides of our brains as fully functioning humans (and this is now totally measurable and is scientifically proven). This is a time when we can both manipulate the

numbers and adroitly design a facade or
paint a painting with totally balanced
skill, comprehension, and control.

So, today, we finally become fully aware
mentally, then we die and vibrationally
start over. Our society loses out in this
process and you do also since you
never reach fruition. Sexually, its as if
we all reached age sixteen then died.

Interestingly, this is why young
architects, who always needed both
sides of their minds, do not yet quite
have it yet. Thus, most of us virtually all
die well before we can take advantage
of our full spiritual and mental resources
years before we can fully access them.
So what great buildings do we miss in
this process? It is true of all of the arts
also: What great paintings have we lost
in this ongoing process?

Today, we worship the youth, those
really ignorant beginners in society, who
do not have a clue how things work yet.
However, for the most part, these are
the only ones who are at all thriving in

our society. The youth are the ones
who still have a reasonable supply of
organic borrowed nutrients from their
mothers and, thus, the stored energy to
thrive on. Add some medium quality oil
based food and they might get by fine
for a few more years, but its going to
run out generally for all in our society by
age fifty or so. For me, it was totally
depleted at age 56.

The few, in our society, who manage to
get to 100 generally have squeaked
past 80 as sickly, shaking, nearly deaf
and blind, and dying. However, these
should be the ones that we should be
emulating, not our youth. They should
be the ones with total resources who are
ready to meet the spiritual, mental, and
physical world in all it has to offer.
However, in fact, almost never is
anyone worth considering among the
very few in that segment today. Sure,
we applaud them just for surviving
against these incredible odds that our
system has handed the hundred year
olds since they have dodged some
serious bullets in getting there.

So we turn to youth, but today, the youth
are also becoming ill at abnormal rates
and this is accelerating also. They are
replete with illnesses that did not exist
just a hundred years ago like Type II
diabetes and, as discussed above,
autoimmune diseases and allergies. So
what awaits us as a society on this path?
Large factory farming and dense city
models create overall sick societies that
cling to life from birth to death with a
very low average quality of life
compared to pre-oil societies,

One last observation on massing people
together as is now encouraged: Just as
our mass shootings demonstrate, it is
far easier to kill a lot of people fast when
they are clumped up, whether it is man
created disaster or a natural one. When
high-rise apartment building fails,
thousands must die. Graham Hancock
offers comments on this.

Teaching Our Minds
Hearing the Right Stuff

So your body with its trillions of
specialized cells is listening carefully
even if you are unaware that you are
talking. The real question is what is what
do you want those cells to hear? First,
the idea is to keep the channels clear
and the conversation loving as Dr.
Lipton teaches. But next, just remember
that they literally hear everything:

When you feel stress, worry, or anger,
you must develop methods that allow
you to let the negatives go quickly and
never dwell on them so as not to put
your cells into an anxiety attack.
Stresses are normal to some degree
and your body can accommodate them,
but only for short spurts. These short
bursts, are no different than climbing a
tree when a lion attacks. They are
coping tools to a point.

After that, they go deep into your body
cells and raise havoc... bad chemistry.
But this is especially bad because your

overall internal chemistry changes with them and stays there till something displaces it or you forget what created the problem in the first place and hopefully move on.

A key point here: when stress, worry, or anger does come. This is not the time to meditate (as many teach), for most people. This is true because, unless you are extremely powerful spiritually, you will likely only take the problem deeper into the sub- consciousness. It normally can take years of spiritual work to be able to handle such things properly, to escape them at the turn of a dime and turn them around. So what do you do?

One way to beat negative emotions is to find an emotion that is even more emotionally interesting to your unconscious self or that is at least as powerful.

So you switch your attention using the above rule: One absolute spiritual rule is that you can only focus consciously on

one emotional issue at a time. Keep
that in mind. So pick a fight with
someone that your rational mind can't
possibly defend (no basis). You have to
really get into this for it to work, then
simply apologize, and walk away.

Another is to fall in love with something
or someone as Dr. Lipton suggests in
his interviews. If you focus on that
person or some difficult problem that
you love, this love can easily transcend
emotions and displace them. Sex is
good, sure, but of course, you do not
want to be taking our basic problems out
on your mate, so be very careful with
this one. Still, good, hard sex is a great
mind clearer for the most part.

Finally, playing a competitive game like
tennis is also a very good way to
refocus and clear your mind of
problems. The key is to clear the mind
first, then Meditate, Contemplate, or
Soul Travel afterwards. Thus, you delve
into the spiritual when you have cleaned
out the cobwebs and are free to travel,
not before, when you can easily take

them deeper into the subconscious
where they can further grab your
subconscious mind.

Long Term Lessons

So where do you want your mind to stop?
Certainly, not on one of the various
mental tie-ups that can consume you
and divert you from love. However,
there are no firm rules here, only
guidelines, tools for you to keep in mind.
Just remember that you have them.

While sex is a useful tool to divert your
mind from all-consuming problems, like
all enjoyable things, when taken too far,
it can, itself, tie you into mental places
that are again all-consuming. So be
careful there. Still, sex is probably the
best and most enjoyable form of
exercise on earth. It not only improves
your physical body, it helps clear out
those mental cobwebs and allows many
things to clear up, as my book, "Pretty
Fine Sex is Spiritual" points this out in
profound ways:

Weight Gain... and Light
A Fresh Look at a Pervasive Problem
Today in the US:

This topic never was very high on my
own personal list till just this year. It all
began when I stopped playing tennis
indoors over the winter and the weather
defined my exercise for the most part
and I switched to peanuts as a snack.
So I gained 15 lbs for the first time in
50 years and my clothes stopped fitting.

As a result, this put my attention, for the
first time, squarely on this great social
problem that is occurring in the US
especially, but also in all developed
countries to some extent.

Seventy percent of your body weight is
the result of sunlight and light (and is
thus directly vibrational and only 30% is
from food which is indirectly vibrational
per the video below (but I find is closer
to 80/20 for me), then you realize just

105

how important the garbage that we buy
in stores is in terms of weight gain and
loss. Most doctors and nutritionists
regard peanuts as decent food, and
occasionally they are, but this
combination for the first time in my life
helped put a belly on me.

When you witness this directly, you
realize just how silly dietary weight loss
programs really are given that my own
diet is, by any standard, exemplary. It is
far better than any advertised or
planned weight loss program that could
possibly be marketed to the public or
actually be sold to make money and I
know exactly the amount in pounds that
I take in per day and here is my story:

I never eat spaghetti, pizza, carbs, any
commercial snacks, sugar, no canned
foods ever, except an occasional
sardine. With this powerful ketogenic,
quantum (microcellular oriented) diet, I
take two heaping tablespoons of MSM a
day. This frees me of all toxins and I
only drink structured "Living Water."

My average mitochondrial cellular count (MC) remains at 2000 and my cellular age is currently 16, so I am not at all within the usual demographics of a 76 year old, or even the most athletic and weight conscious segment of US society that could likely come close to posting these numbers. A normal, exceptional 76 year old has 500 (MC) maximum mitochondria per cell and their normal cellular age, in the US, today is 200MC by our testing and an average 16 year old is 1000MC.

However, a few years ago I got a very accurate set of scales and started monitoring my weight gain and loss, which, till this year, was nailed at 146 lbs. Mind you that my weight on leaving Air Force boot camp at 19 was 142. I had just gained twenty pounds in eight weeks. I came out of boot camp weighing ten pounds less than I do today at 151. Only last year, my weight dropped to 142 and I started paying more attention to my weight. My clothes were falling off. So this started with more than a 10% weight gain in one year... huge for me.

With the above strict diet, I lightly exercise, playing doubles tennis every other day on average. As we hear, exercise changes our metabolic rates. But I stopped exercise for two winter months and my weight went to an astounding 157 pounds and my clothes were too small! So today, I am holding at a 10% gain. But the less obvious thing was the jar of peanuts on my desk... a deadly combination with no exercise had to go.

Now here is my point: By https://www.youtube.com/watch?v=mOQ2SmaDLOY (4:55 is a key point here, but there is a lot more here of value). Our main source of energy from the mitochondria is the 570 to 850 NM light range per this video. Obviously, few are getting it. Given this, what you eat is far less important than your vibrational sources for body weight, but there are other factors.

Given the above: I have a well defined and carefully planned diet that allows me to monitor why and how my body weight changes. Here are some facts that I have carefully measured:

- Just with sleep, my weight commonly drops 3 to 5 pounds and I eat much less in food than this weight loss can explain. So this is what it takes to dream (run your mind and body). My food intake is 1/4 lb. average per day, but may go as high as 1/2 lb. maximum and I just never paid much attention to intake amounts. With commonly considered science and nutrition, this weight gain makes no sense.

- My total water plus food intake is 7 1/4 lbs. a day. Of that 7 lbs is our structured "Living Water." I am 100% hydrated at all times by test. Interestingly, I am simply never hungry or thirsty and have not been in years, so the peanuts were always a habit. Finally, my own energy

input from food is much less than
20%.

As the above video points out almost
none of this is related to food intake.

I do eat an occasional small orange,
that helps with my MSM (organic C), so
a little fructose and what my garden
gives me in season.

The point here is that my stopping
winter tennis and a few peanuts had a
dramatic effect on my weight and I
cannot be exceptional in this way. This
has to be true for all of us. Within seven
days of starting my tennis, with Spring,
and dropping the peanuts, my weight
dropped from 157 to 151 . Now, it is
holding steady at 148. Nothing about
my diet otherwise or my water intake
has changed. My clothes still do not fit
correctly, so I must lose 4 more pounds
or buy new ones soon.

In doing this, for the first time, I finally
realize just how unscientific and how far
off these popular weight reduction

programs are from reality. Also, how closely tied our metabolic rate can be to light exercise and bad snacks.

This should be a very important pointer for people who actually have weight problems and, if you are one of them with excess fat, these observations should give you some idea of what you are up against with mainstream advice. It is simply not about cutting back on portions or excessively exercising, but here are some generalities:

- If your diet is perfect, you can easily gain 10% in body weight by slowing down your metabolic rates just from not getting exercise. If my body can change this much, under these conditions, so can yours.

- On the opposite side, if your diet consists of sugars and carbohydrates, how much more could you add to my 10%? I eat none

- Food quality, in general, for me, has not changed, so this has no perceptible affect on body weight. It is all about keeping my metabolism up with mild exercise and no snacks. That is, exercise is tennis with some gardening and pushing a power mower. But these last pounds, are going to take awhile, now that they are here and my body has latched onto this new form as I discuss.

- Fasting: I only fast for 24 hours, but so far, no effect.

- Low E glass, universal in today's high efficiency windows, reduces the available spectrum of sunlight just as LED bulbs do, but without the blue problems. So Dr. Mercola does not have the whole story as he assumes.
  https://www.thermalwindows.com/products/lowe/

- Daylighting: Windows do not admit full spectrum lighting. Nothing beats direct sunlight (a food) outside at noon for full spectrum healthy lighting. In more northern climates, you must supplement with vitamin D3 accordingly in winter.

- Artificial lighting: Keep in mind that halogen is the best, most energy efficient in avoiding LED's, but low voltage DC is by far the best full spectrum lighting source.

- We are quantum beings: The above serves to prove that the entire medical and building world have both lost sight of the fact of who we are. Our body assumes a shape according to all it anticipates, but It is all happening at the mitochondrial level in ways that cannot be measured, anticipated, or understood by today's science.

- The human body re-corrects and assumes a shape that it accepts as best to survive, thus changing that assumption is the major issue here. Once it takes that form, it assumes and holds that shape as correct.

- Today's science looks at your body as a simple heat engine... calories in and calories out. This is why our society as a whole keeps getting bigger in size and is dreadfully undernourished. Your body knows a shape If your diet changes, it may give up weight to go to that shape, but changing that will take a lot.

- Until the scientific model changes, things are not going to reverse and no fad diet will ever fix things.

Foods To Avoid

https://www.youtube.com/watch?v=dTieMc72eZs
If you want to train your body to use the correct foods, you must avoid the following foods: grains and cultured rice, sugar and even too much fruit, but no

bananas, peanuts, cashews, or cooked
nuts, dried beans, kidney beans,
bread, pasta, potatoes or high Lectin
foods, large fish, and anything raised in
or from bad soils with chemicals.
However, the list goes on and I have
given you plenty of clues. Still, it begins
with a low carb, Keto diet. Seldom if
you follow the reasoning behind all of
this will you feel restricted and I never
feel hungry or thirsty after over ten years.

UVB sunlight is a food (just as LED
(blue) lighting is a bad food) and the
above associated products consumed
for any length of time will cause weight
gain and related problems. However,
with me it was light exercise and no
snacking on peanuts, a high Lectin food.
With these, I noticed small, but
immediate changes.

Herbs
Amazing Supervegetables

So earlier, I introduced you to the
vegetables that you eat maybe with

every meal. Here, I list some of the
various amazing herbs that can change
various aspects of your life in ways that
few are aware can occur. First, I
referenced this information from the
"Lost Empire" sales website and you
can get plenty more information if you
go there. I have used some of them for
many years, but a few are totally new to
me. However, it is well known that
various herbs have been doing their
jobs for years and are below is my short
list, but when you are hurting or have a
special condition, the can fill-in needs
that you are missing:

- Triphala, an Ayuvedic Herb, is a
  mixture of three: Haritaki,
  Bhibitaki, and Amalaki. It has
  been a celebrated mix in India for
  thousands of years. It aids in
  nearly every aspect of wellness
  and especially food absorption
  and antioxidant content.

- Shatavari, known as Asparagus
  Racemosus, is a long regarded
  herb, and one I recommend when

our own gardens are not
producing the good stuff.

- He Shou Wu, the antiaging herb
for those who do not quite get
this book down quite as well as
they would wish they did.

- Rhodiola Rosea, was brought
back by the USSR to benefit their
athletes, but its great for mental
function and clarity. It is great for
tennis players and it is noticeable
if you are paying attention.

- Nettle Root, the stuff grows
about everywhere and if it has
stung you, you will remember
what it is, but it's great for most
every American male over sixty
given our terrible diets. We have
a general population with
enlarged prostates by that age. It
should not happen, but it does.
Also, it aids in sexual dysfunction
and limits DHT. But read the
precautions please.

- Mecuna Purens, has long been on my list as a full spectrum health supplement and it does give both sexes a nice boost while it calms.

- Maca, yes, but eat this stuff as food not an herb as I presented earlier and more is better. It repairs and protects your brain among other things as I report.

- Lions Mane, mushroom for the brain. A memorable herb for sure.

- Seabuckthorn, I have been taking this herb off and on for many years for its immune system enhancements, but there are plenty of other qualities assigned to it. Most unique of them is it stops tooth decay. So can kids still eat their candy when they take it?

- Muira Puama (Horny Goat Weed, is not hard to sell, since our

culture is a mess sexually. Use it
with care.

- Tongkat Ali, is probably better
  than the above, long-term, for
  men's sex and with no down-side.
  Additionally, T. Ali could help get
  that six-pack back.

- Cordyceps, this most expensive
  herb on the planet, is not really a
  mushroom, but it has many good
  things going for it and is most
  likely an antiaging herb also
  along with He Shu Wu.

- Tribulus Terrestris, a very hardy
  plant that survives in very dry
  locations. Is useful for kidney,
  bladder, and urinary tract health.
  It is a testosterone enhancer in
  males and increases glucose and
  lipid profiles in diabetics.

- Butea Supurba has been found to
  increase sexual enhancement
  and blood flow. It contains
  flavinoids and steroid compounds.

- Tongkat Ali (Longjac), a Malaysian tree, cleans estrogen receptors and may offer some protection against breast cancer. It is a holistic energy booster and sexual enhancer for both sexes. Use in small amounts 400mg @ 1:100 extract two days, then skip a day. It always enhances stamina and blood flow. It is dry, spicy, and bitter. It can be dissolved in water. It is greasy and almost black in color.

- Ziziphus, is most likely a better long-term choice than melatonin as a sleep aid and with no down-side. It is the top Chinese choice for that. Take it with GABA... read the methylation cycles to see why.

The above could obviously be the topic of many new books and studies. Herbs alone could easily take up lifetimes of intensive research. However, if you are serious about stopping your aging and staying well, you need to learn all you can about herbs. They are, as you would expect, intensely vibratory.

Why We Die From the Physical Point of View

Recall that often you hear of people dying of natural causes. The term normally is used to describe a death from disease as opposed to an accident or a murder. But illness is not natural to our bodies and, like death, it really is a form of agreement. This agreement may between you and the government or only within your mind. But death is always a form of agreement. An accidental death, on some level, is an agreement, even if we are not aware that we have made it. "Death from Old Age:" was once a common term. Now if a coroner put that statement on a death certificate, he would likely lose his job.

Our agreement: As we know, when a spouse dies, the other often follows quickly, especially in what we now term

"old age." That is, we have agreed to
live within a term that we consider
normal and when a loving spouse dies
within that term, we simply follow from
stress. When that happens, as we see,
it often takes very little time. This
because we have already agreed to die
within a certain time frame. Even a
minor upset, under those conditions can
stop a beating heart. Is that death from
"old age?" Under these conditions, yes.

The basic point of this book is that no
one can die of "old age." First, you must
find ways to age and these after a
certain maturity are not even normal.
Then you must find a way to die. We
assume that we will age and certainly,
we are not going to stay babies or even
teenagers. And we must reach a degree
of maturity, but after a point, we can
reach a level of equalization and
balance. This is the point where we no
longer actually age if we find the correct
mix of antioxidants and oxidants to keep
us within a range of stability. Today, that
point is just never reached in our society

The Bottom Line here is that we must learn to love all of life and not be totally dependent on anyone. This degree of independence does not take away love, but adds to it.

As a spiritual being this is the greatest contribution that you can make to life. It is not limiting, but is expanding. With this, you become the God person that you are entitled to be.

Drug Warnings

Why you are warned not to take a drug when you have:

- "Serious infections:" A serious infection will turn on your body's autoimmune system. Drugs are designed to steal from and thus compromise your autoimmunity. If your autoimmunity were operating perfectly, you would never find the need for a drug, since you would never have a health condition. However, it is because drugs can trade off conditions that they actually, to some degree, work and why they nearly always bring side effects. If you autoimmune system is already activated by a "serious infection," the drug can easily confuse (borrow from) your defense system, thus making that infection worse. Also, chances are, the drug will never work at all during a "serious infection," so you are warned not to take it then.

- "If you have Heart Disease or Cancer" (life threatening diseases that activate the autoimmune system). This is a redundant warning similar to "Serious infection", but a drug that steals from your autoimmune system when you have a life threatening disease just might be enough to put your body over the edge and kill you under the wrong conditions and this happens often enough, but seldom is reported.

- "If you are pregnant or plan to be":
  You read how the fetus steals
  nutrients in any way necessary
  so it can survive. That being the
  case, you sure do not want a
  drug compromising your system
  on top of this biological load.
  There are a minute few drugs
  that use some natural means to
  alter your system and these need
  not carry this warning.

What is a drug? Obviously, if any
organic food were discovered by a
drug company and it happened to be
unique enough to be allowed a
patent, it would be termed a drug
and then become too expensive to
eat. Drugs are first-off patented,
mainly as tradeoffs to natural ways
of doing things, but commonly are
pieces of them.

Fortunately for us: Maringa, coconut
oil, green beans, asparagus and
maca likely cannot ever be patented
or they would be beyond the reach of

most of us and no drug on earth will
ever equal them in pure organic form.
But the above are not tradeoffs, they
are organic lines of defense that can
complement the autoimmune system.

So listen and laugh with me when you
hear the drug ads and the drug
warnings that must, by law, follow them.
The dirt on any organic food is that it far
surpasses anything that can manipulate
your brilliant autoimmune system. Given
the proper tools, no matter what your
chronological age, your body can out
maneuver diseases. But, keep in mind
that even a brand new car will falter if it
has no gas in its tank.

The Vibrations of Life
Spiritual Transformations
All of life has been driven by vibrations
since the beginning of time and I have
written on this often. They begin as
sound, but transform into light. As a
human being, Soul (chose your term),
has the ability to capture and hold them
within the pituitary, the seat of Soul,
where they radiate and transform all or

your cells. Thus, you are, as Soul, a
package of vibrations that happens to
take a human body to learn love.

This is why you are here and why you
may be allowed to stay longer than we
are presently allocated in this dance of
life. But it is why you may be forced to
move on before you think you are ready.
You do get to vote, but if you are not
learning love at the rate you should be,
you will move on, even if you are
kicking and screaming.

If you are paying attention, this "Sound
of God," which varies according to the
vibratory level or spiritual plane that we
are placing our attention on, is always
there. But this sound is now a proven
measurable scientific fact as reported in
my last book. Furthermore, when your
attention is raised to a higher level, the
sound (and associated light) changes
tune. This sound is captivating and
beautiful in each of its forms. Once you
have experienced this consciously, this
sound is quite dramatic and it affects
everything in your life and you can
reinitiate it with contemplation (chose

your term), bringing it back into your
awareness.

When you get this, you have earned it.
You own it, but it does not come easily.
Since this process is so all-transforming,
spirit generally serves it up gradually,
but this is not always the case either.
Occasionally, it comes like a flash of
lightening that simply transforms and
changes everything... an awakening.
When this occurs, it generally can take
years to readjust; still, it is a wonderful
gift.

The doctors above are reporting from
levels that just do not teach us this stuff.
However, with their new awareness,
they do teach chanting and spirituality
that only in the recent past was totally
off topic in science and what they say is
indeed transforming. It has been a long
time coming, yet it is being embraced
again even by many scientists after a
long hiatus.

However, the topic here begins beyond
the unconscious, which they term the

automatic mind. But before going there, let's be clear that the levels beyond the unconscious allow us to reprogram the unconscious to what we agree to and not what we were taught up to age seven as Lipton and science teaches. The point is that we can indeed know all levels once we pass into the 5th dimension in full awareness.

Furthermore, when we make this transformation into the 5th plane and beyond, all of the cells in our bodies are transformed with us and others with this level of awareness see this light emanating as visible light. When you see them recognize it, there are no doubts. We share the 5th plane or higher.

Finally, not all Souls enter their body as beginners as Dr. Lipton suggests in his talks. In fact, a few advanced Soul's recall past lives (vibrations) to the degree that they are totally aware immediately on birth. In the case of my friend Fran, she took the body of a three year old when that child fell out of a

three story window. When Fran B.
recovered from that fall, she was the
high level spiritual being that she was
prior to the fall, but in full awareness.
This is, of course, very unusual, but
there are endless possibilities spiritually.

In my own case, I was highly aware
from age one on. My main chore on
birth was to readjust to this realm. Thus,
I can recall every important spiritual
event from birth and I was simply not
programmed by anyone. I programmed
myself and still do it consciously. Most
all of my dream life is spent working with
others, healing them, mostly spiritually.
Occasionally, I am allowed to help
someone cross over and avoid the
intimidating Angel of Death... a very
special and loving adventure.

My most wonderful of those occurred
with my brother Steve when he died in
2017. Generally, one must be a 9th to
do this, so I was given this initiation to
allow it. So Steve avoided that Angel of
Death and when he crossed, he knew
just what he was getting and he was

ecstatic about what he saw ahead of him. Today, I keep his picture on my computer screen to remind me to touch base with him daily. No one could be happier than he is in the place he consciously chose and he was very picky.

What usually happens: The real dirt is that the Angel of Death just looks at you. In that instant, It knows just where you are spiritually and you are assigned your new place based on what you have earned, period. It could be here on earth or on a higher plane according to what we need. There is no bargaining here, and it can be very scary, but you get what you earn without question.

Forget what religions teach on this topic. I have actually observed this happening and it simply is not much fun, but its always fair and loving in its outcome. No matter what you are taught or how well you have lived by your religious rules, you will stand before this entity and be judged unless you are led beyond it and few ever are.

Brother Steve was very fortunate to have bypassed this process and be given this opportunity and he knows it. His is a choice spot on the 3rd plane. These assignments are always temporary, but he picked a very cool place and he loves it as most any anyone would... It is beautiful! I was very fortunate to have been able to accompany him in finding it. The most fun thing about it was in how very careful and meticulous he was in selecting his place. This literally took all night, moving at light speed!

Below I will discuss some specialized physical transformations that we can all go through, but love is the key and these are certainly not the point of your existence:

Breath Control: Breath is a voluntary manifestation up to a point. The point here is that you can take breath control to a point where you can hook this voluntary function "breath" to involutary functions such as heart beat and

basically all normally involuntary bodily
functions such as heart beat, blood
pressure, digestion, the release of
hormones, and at the microcellular level,
energy release. For women, they can
relatively easily alter menstral release
and duration. There are useful
applications for all of these and of
course, they throw wrenches into all
medical testing when mainstream tests
are used. After all, what good is a pulse
rate when you can voluntarily make it
half the normal rate?

Breatharians, who are doing these
things to an extreme, prove their control
in this one case, avoid food and water;
https://www.youtube.com/watch?v=XyN
9Eh04QPU My point here is that we can
learn from the extreme, take them into
balance, and use them in ways that are
controlled.

All involuntary body systems can learn
from the voluntary. menstrual cycles
are now considered involuntary. One
obvious proof that women can alter their
menstrual cycles is that in an office.

environment they all commonly involuntarily cycle together. This is one aspect of changing involuntarily cycles and it proves that you can do it. Now consider that you can change any system that is arwy including diseases as discussed earlier through the release of, "letting go of", that is trying to control, your mind.

I am not saying that the path to total wellness is through the extreme practice of giving up food as with the above "breatharian" practice. However, you are never going to become totally well until you back off from our extreme lack of self control and discipline in today's spoon fed society.

The "Small House"

Everything that we have discussed up till this point is illustrates high performance, well organized methods: Our yards, our meals, etc. What we are always discussing, though, is density. Density imples extreme quality, organic methods and considerations, using science, but with low technology. This effort should not stop with our yards, our water, or our food. It certainly extends to our living spaces which can affect our health in profound ways. Our building materials today outgas chemicals and our lighting, as discussed below and previously, has profound health affects, but there is much more to consider.

The Concept: I cut my teeth in architecture with passive solar design. This solar design (basically forgotten today even though it is still far better than photovoltaics or wind solutions) taught that a house performed with the sun just as our bodies do, so the house, properly designed, becomes a refined solar collector, itself, just as your body is.

Therefore, a house that uses heat in winter should collect and store solar energy: Whether you design it to specifically do that or not, all houses perform according to their solar orientation, prevailing wind, and local

storm resistance and no one today
seems to get this simple fact.

Interestingly, a house that is correctly
laid out and oriented is generally
cheaper to build per unit volume, it stays
cooler in summer and may even heat
itself in winter Long term, such a house
is far cheaper to own and it is a lovely
place to inhabit. But the overall first cost
here is also often much less than
conventional tract houses simply
because it wastes no space. Also, long
term, it maintains itself well using natural
materials when intelligently employed.

The basic layout: The first criteria for
system performance is to locate the day
time living spaces on the south side.
You would like your kitchen on the east
to wake up with the rising sun and
certainly any guest bedrooms on the
north where they buffer that cold wall.
Garages are best detached in today's
world, since cars today do not really
require heating. But either way, the
garage should buffer the house from
weather and never be on the south..

The Spa Room: With our knowledge of
DMSO and the healing qualities of salt
water, there should be a hot tub room
on the south side that is mostly heated
passively by sunlight, but also by lost
heat from the hot tub *hot water solar?"
Preferably, the salt water would be
trucked-in from a clean off-shore ocean
source, if this is feasible, but otherwise,
the salt would come from clean ancient
salt deposits and contain plenty of
minerals. This should also include a
Sauna and it should be very cozy and a
very sexy place to hang out.

Living spaces, generally, should be fairly
small by today's standards, but they
should be designed for both high quality
sound and video. Soon, with advent of
quantum computing and video, expect
new volume requirements for any sitting
space that will make most living rooms
extinct. But for now, this should be a
volume space to take this into account
this technology evolves later (it is on its
way now) and they are adapted.

Now I include a layout for a house with this fixed plan, but obviously, there are infinite variations even with the pieces that I give you. One of the problems with 99% of the houses today is that they are almost never designed by professionals even when builders claim that they are.

The idea in today's world is that a draftsmen or carpenter can do a good enough job designing and that saves first-cost fees, so builders can be more competitive. The market likes oversize spaces (waste) and they sell well for builders. The contrary suggestion here is that design quality saves space and finished space is expensive. Nothing wastes money faster than poorly designed excess finished space.

Finally, the selected design professional should understand all building systems and be extremely capable in heating, ventilation, plumbing, and air conditioning and especially be adept at working on very small scales. Distribution (ducting) is not a key element here, but it should be oversize

for the most part, with low air volume
movement (cfm's).

Built-in, not bought furniture: here, a
bedroom as just that, a platform space
for a mattress, and it should be tight,
mirrored, and very sexy with no added
furniture, such as a dressing table or
chest of drawers. This should all be built
into the closet and the Living Area.

A bedroom should include a roof
window that can be completely shut off
from light and EM frequencies as much
as possible, but still allow two people to
look at the stars at appropriate times
and also allow self-ventilation and to
wake up with the birds seasonally with
forced ventilation and cooling as
appropriate. Thus, should be climate
controlled separately from the house as
much as possible for a small space but
it may draw air from the larger space.

The house should include a well
equipped exercise room near the hot tub
room.

There should be plenty of closet space
(cheap) with simple built-in shelves and
dressing areas. The baths (expensive)
need not be too big, since we have a hot
tub room (expensive) ,so just showers.
The hot tub room also serves as birthing
room, by the way, and water
temperatures should be digitally touch
controlled with a fast response time.

We want this house to not only
accommodate exercise, but it must be
inverted so that we must use the stairs
to get to those sexy, cool but very cozy,
living spaces upstairs. This also allows
for sitting decks which also are good
emergency egressways in the event of a
fire with sliding doors (rather than
egress windows).

So the bottom line here is that our
houses are too big and most are
incredibly badly designed, dangerous in
some ways, and wasteful in virtually
every way. We applaud them as
healthy and safe, just as we do our drug
and food industries.

In fact, our building codes implement
and encourage this level of waste today.
Poor design is often even enforced in
certain ways, but any good design
professional can slip past their
ignorance. As this book points out, the
direction that our lighting design is going
is wrong and will become more enforced
and become worse.

The diagrams that I show you are two
Bedroom (BR) upstairs and one finished
BR downstairs with a total downstairs
finished area of 1340 sf and upstairs
area of 650, so less than 2000 square
feet of finished living space. This
translates into less than $300,000 in
most less dense locations (at $150/sf
finished space), not cities, of course.

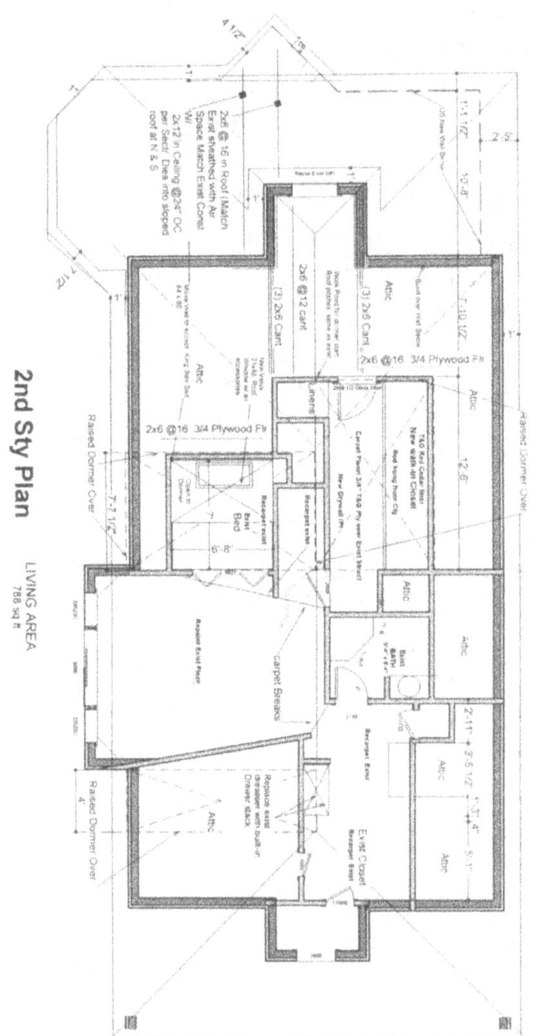

142

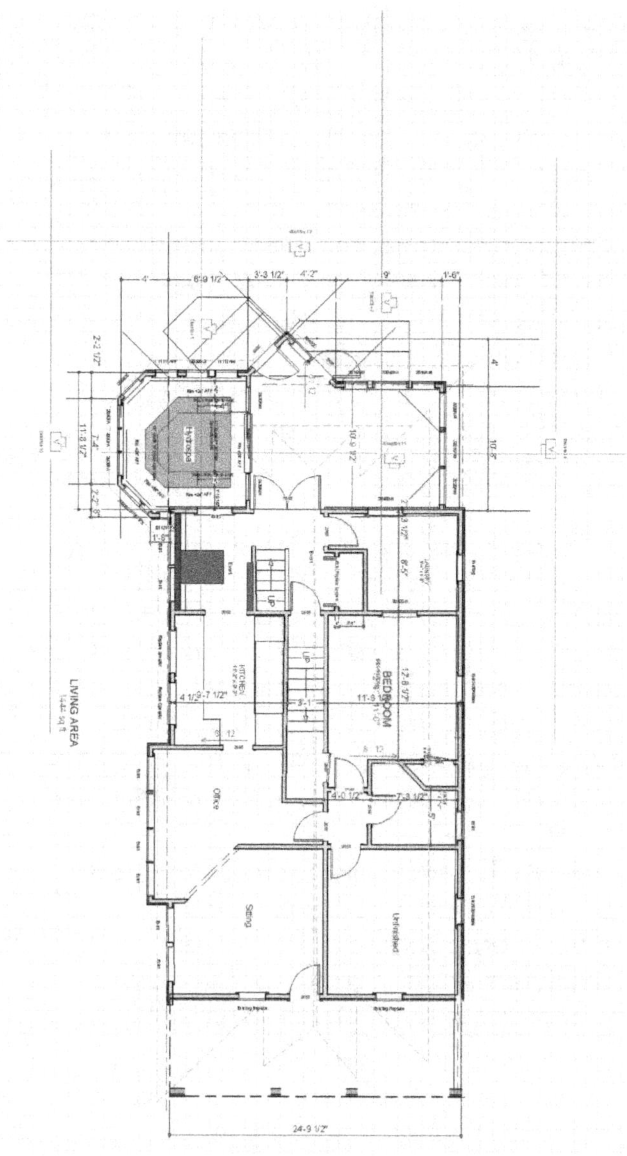

143

https://www.youtube.com/watch?v=GIJK
3dwCWCw
These plans were a part of a set of
technical drawings and specifications.
They are not presentation drawings, but
the diagrams meet the above criteria for
a house that does all that is outlined in
the "Small House" and any good
Architect can get my intentions from
them. Seldom in today's world does
anyone any one even know enough to
request this level of design
sophistication.

This particular house was designed for
the 38th parallel so it has that shape
factor. Conversely, and the DOE proved
this, the ideal house on the equator is
round and on the 50th latitude is
stretched out to a 3 to 1 shape factor.
So you see, from this, a house conforms
to its latitude as well as local weather.

Eventually, when quantum computers
are completely understood and
developed, houses will become
intelligent enough to adapt their outer
shape to the sun. So the shape factor

will adapt to the solar conditions at that time of day and its latitude. With this level of sophistication, you will speak to your house as you do a pet today and it will learn your particular needs.

Till that time comes, our houses must be designed to manually alter their responses to outer conditions. Interestingly, the most sophisticated way of doing that today is still with low tech, thousand-year old Venetian blinds. We have changed their composition and made them wider and narrower according to fads, but they are still the best solution to sun control and heat loss that we have.

Looking Young

So we, herein, have discussed virtually every important aspect of antiaging and, generally, what it takes to get there. While these key elements all begin at the microcellular level as discussed previously, there are options at the dermal level that work in conjunction

with these microcellular functions.
However, the claims that one can
happen without the other, at least long
term is bogus. Spreading on beauty
creams topically without attacking the
true problem is like painting a house
with rotten cedar siding. Wellness and
youth are systemic.

I nearly brought out a skin cream when I
wrote my first book. The ingredients of
such a cream are obvious, but despite
the "scientific" claims of commercial
creams, before and after pictures are
temporary and bogus. I will run through
some of the science and you can
formulate a far more effective treatment
system and cream than you can buy
anywhere. Maybe, at some point, I will
formulate the system as I planned.
Today, I still have my original "Orange
Cream" in a jar that I apply after a
shower as a system..

To begin, before you apply any cream,
you should apply some amount of
DMSO. I apply that at 100% strength to
my entire face and exposed skin

including my closed eye lids,. Before going there, do some testing though. I need not remind you that we are all different. DMSO can go through the eyelids and improve vision, but before that, it will hydrate skin and remove wrinkles around your eyes.

One thing that you will discover in doing this is that if you use one finger to apply it, that finger will wrinkle up just as your fingers do when you take a very long bath. This, it over-hydrates that finger print the same way.

Now hopefully in reading the last chapter you caught the idea of using a Salt Water/ DMSO hot tub and if you do not have one yet, it is on your wish list, because these two things are absolutely hydrating and there is no topical cream on earth that can equal its transdermal hydrating effects. For a more in depth discussion, read Chapter 46 in "It's the Liver Stupid," but I will review some of the key elements below:

Topical nutrients: The use of
transdermal magnesium in that hot tub
is key here. Magnesium relaxes
everything, including the skin and
muscles that support it. If I were making
up a skin lotion some form of organic
Magnesium would be included. Next,
the magic orange nutrient Astaxanthin is
a key nutrient. Cilantro and chlorella
tinctures are excellent for a few weeks
at a time. So you see, our cream is best
varied over time.

Exfoliation is a key component here also.
with this, you are literally sanding off the
older top layer. You can do it with a buff
puff daily or a plastic surgeon can do it
all at once for you and make your life
unbearable for several days. His dermal
abrasion may be very uncomfortable,
but you should read my first book to see
the ingredients in commercial creams
that are sold to make your skin better
and some are carcinogens. With skin
cancer, you could ruin a great deal more
than just a few weeks of your time.

The final key here is that "Looking Young" is a process, not a face saving application just as what is occurring within at the cellular level and all places in between, so be patient and take small steps. This book advocates a very long and enjoyable lifetime with plenty of love.

The Wrap on Dirt

So herein, I have pointed our many factors that cause us to age. Aging, of course, is a long-term experiment that will go on till we graduate to the timeless 5th plane where Soul takes over. Here, I focus on what I consider to be some profound facts that are seldom, if ever, expressed today by even the most profound health advisors. I have pointed out some facts that you can test in casual conversations with your friends and, obviously, try yourself to whatever degree you wish. I have also pointed out why your contribution to life can be much more profound if you choose this simple course and not just follow what the mainstream and your government has in store for you. Nothing that they know of on earth will ever surpass the unpatented, low-tech "Dirt" that you were born with.

Cheers, Jim

Videography/ Bibliography:

For videos that document, explain, prove, but mostly complement this book, search: You Tube/ James Robert Clark Quantum Science or cut and paste the following URLs:
CP4U, a QM device as used in a car (our first application):
https://www.youtube.com/watch?v=YFakNUEQoNM
https://www.youtube.com/watch?v=LcWN_DSmlAl
Life Extension Results
https://www.youtube.com/watch?v=DAQ_sdcgaBM
Potential Lifespan
https://www.youtube.com/watch?v=eH_wcdu2u-4
https://www.youtube.com/watch?v=06kXgs00Cxw

An Introduction to Spontaneous Evolution" Bruce H. Lipton, PhD

"Back Hole" Nassim Haramein

"Beyond Pyramid Power," Dr. Patrick Flanagan, PhD
ISBN 0-87516-208-8

"The Biology of Belief" Bruce H. Lipton, PhD
https://www.brucelipton.com/books/biology-of-belief

"White Paper" Dan Nelson, PhD
Https://www.waybackwater.com/dans-white-paper

Books below by James Robert Clark addressing health available at Amazon books:
"It's The Liver Stupid," 5th edition/ Video Ref
        Paperback: 324 pages
    Platform; 5th edition (11/19/17)
        ISBN-13: 978-1547010493"Beyond Epigenetics" Paperback 120 Pages   Platform 1st Edition   ISBN   "Methylation, Awareness and You"
        Print Length: 114 pages
        Platform; 2nd edition
Publication Date: December 19, 2014

BASIN: B00R8P7R3   ISBN-13: 978-1981214280
  "Between the Jeans"
  (a complete rewrite of the Above Book)
   SBN-13: 978-1981214280
    Publication Date: Nov 17,2017
  Platform: 1st edition
  114 Pages
  Paperback
  Platform 1st Edition/ Video Ref
  "Pretty Fine Sex is Spiritual"
  Paperback 182 pages
  Platform 1st Edition
  ISBN-13 978 1495396741

  "Your Better Half"
  The art of the ART
  124 Pages
  Paperback
  Platform: 1st Edition
  Publication Date: Feb 8 2018
   ISBN-13 978-1985205321
  124 Pages
  Paperback

Videography

Graham Hancock is interviewed
regarding ancient suppressed
civilizations 2018
https://www.youtube.com/results?search_query=https%
3A%2F%2Fwww.youtube.com%2Fwatch%3Fv%3DlRPGq
UdkLdw
Howard Garrett, "The Dirt Doctor,"

Dr. Joel Wallach, humorist/ veterinarian
2018 talk
https://www.youtube.com/watch?v=kihm0QMpYCY

Dr. Dan Nelson, 2011 talk "Wayback
Water:"
https://www.youtube.com/watch?v=7hNW7qxlMzg&t=9s

Dr. Bruce Lipton, 2018 Radio Interview
on "Vaccinations," Green Planetfm.com
https://www.youtube.com/watch?v=7QxaG9Ng0ls

Dr. Bruce Lipton May 17, 2017 "Being
Sick is a Hoax"
https://www.youtube.com/watch?v=7wlaViS9EsQ

Drs. Mercola and Wunsch, Oct 18,18
"Dangers of LED Lights"
https://www.youtube.com/watch?v=mOQ2SmaDLOY